Cell Level Meditation

"Written with both poetry and precision, *Cell Level Meditation* synthesizes many ways of knowing and makes very complex material both accessible and fascinating. And it contains the wisdom garnered through years of authentic experience."
— **Julia Brayshaw, M.A.,** psychotherapist, mental health counselor, and author of *Medicine of Place*

"Within the pages of this book, I was delighted to find an elegantly simple offering that guides the reader to a threshold of inner truth through meditation. If you are on a road to discovering true self, Cell Level Meditation is a wonderful point of interest to explore. I am sure you will find the inner view of you to be astounding."
— **Peggy Smith,** certified vibrational medicine practitioner

"*Cell Level Meditation* is a lively narrative that moves between macro and micro, from personal to global—a written expression of the expanding and compressing practice of returning to breath. A deep exploration into our bodies' most basic cellular structures, as well as how we might fit in as cells of a larger cosmos, is pragmatically demonstrated throughout the text in the consistent practice of return to the vital function of breath. In fact, the book breathes!"
— **Dianne Miller,** homeopathic master clinician (HMC)

"This book speaks in an easy way about something incredibly complex. In this beautiful simplicity, it can be read on several levels. By reading it again and again, the process can take you to deeper experiences of awareness for a more profound embodiment. It's a book to hold and return to throughout your journey."
— **Joleen Kelleher,** registered nurse, certified classical homeopath (CCH), and founder of Light Institute for Health

D1554393

"*Cell Level Meditation* evokes in one a desire to reach in and explore sound, breath, visual scapes and fields, and encounters with new horizons that make up its power into levels of potential healing; it beckons and engages. Throughout, it dances into the joy and power of letting the reader in on the healing course that cells are being redirected by Cell Level Meditation and breath. In the closing chapters the reader is gently prodded to 'Go sit in your cell and your cell will teach you everything.' And it further states 'whatever you can imagine, opens possibilities that can burst into physical reality. The noble cells of your body can rest, take stock of the situation, and create solutions to problems. What makes the cells of the body so successful is their ability to cooperate! Sounds like we should be taking classes from them.' One can conclude *Cell Level Meditation* is therefore a companion textbook, a new friend in introducing cell level listening. You'll find the harmonics insightful."

— **Jose Saïd Osio,** publisher, Sacred Passages Death Doula, and educator in the death literacy movement

CELL LEVEL
MEDITATION
The Healing Power in the
Smallest Unit of Life

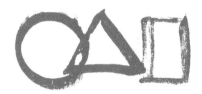

Barry Grundland, M.D.
& Patricia Kay, M.A., CCH, CSD

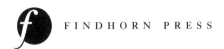 FINDHORN PRESS

Findhorn Press
One Park Street
Rochester, Vermont 05767
www.findhornpress.com

Findhorn Press is a division of Inner Traditions International

Originally published in 2009 by Simply Wonder, LLC, under the title *Cell Level Meditation: Breathing with the Wisdom and Intelligence of the Cell.*
This revised and expanded edition published in 2021 by Findhorn Press.

Disclaimer
The information in this book is given in good faith and is neither intended to diagnose any physical or mental condition nor to serve as a substitute for informed medical advice or care. Please contact your health professional for medical advice and treatment. Neither author nor publisher can be held liable by any person for any loss or damage whatsoever which may arise from the use of this book or any of the information therein.

Cataloging-in-Publication data for this title is available from the Library of Congress

ISBN 978-1-64411-224-3 (print)
ISBN 978-1-64411-225-0 (ebook)

Printed and bound in the United States by Versa Press, Inc.

10 9 8 7 6 5 4 3 2 1

Edited by Michael Hawkins
Text design and layout by Richard Crookes
This book was typeset in Adobe Garamond Pro
Brush painting by Sengai (reversed for the Western mind), Japan, c. 1830, Mitsu Art Gallery, Tokyo.

To send correspondence to the author of this book, mail a first-class letter to the author c/o Inner Traditions • Bear & Company, One Park Street, Rochester, VT 05767, USA and we will forward the communication, or contact the author directly at **www.CellLevelMeditation.com**.

We dedicate this book
to all who have done this work,
as well as to all who will.

Contents

Foreword

I live with my family: my daughter Rikki, son-in-law Simon, and eight-year-old grandson Adam. At 74 I am still practicing law, and my special education clients were all in crises. I had to respond to them as well as follow the latest Department of Education edicts pertaining to their special services. I'm fortunate that my office is in an extra bedroom of my house.

Since March 19th I had been experiencing odd off-and-on-again fevers, but nothing that matched a Covid-19 diagnosis. I had mild fevers every night, mostly 99, and they all vanished during the day. No chest pain, cough, or flu-like symptoms. I had been treated for an unrelenting sinus infection since January and figured those symptoms had morphed.

But that weekend I could not focus; none of the normal legal-ese I have mastered made sense. Then I couldn't get out of bed and began sleeping more.

On March 26th, my concerned daughter insisted I go to the hospital. It took me an hour to get dressed. At the hospital she explained to the techs that I have only one lung from lung cancer; have had a mastectomy and assorted other illnesses that put me in the high Covid risk category. They immediately put a mask on me and wheeled me into an air-tight room. I received a nasal swab and an x-ray.

Surprise! I had pneumonia. I was told I would be kept in the room until the Covid test returned, in 12 hours. Then I recalled that pneumonia is associated with Covid and panic joined me for the endless hours ahead of me. What could I possibly do to protect myself, body-mind-and-spirit?

I immediately recalled Patricia Kay, my life-saver-guide-angel, who ten years before had reached out to help me through a horrid time of being diagnosed with both breast and lung cancer in the same month. A year later I reached out to her again when I was informed the breast cancer had metastasized into a supraclavicular lymph node above the diseased breast. My oncologist told me, with tears in her eyes, that this was a dire prognosis.

But let me start back in September 2010, when Patricia reached out to me from a continent away when she read about my diagnosis in an Integral online group, we both participated in. I am a spiritually inclined yet solidly practical woman, and I wondered how I would deal with a dual diagnosis of primary breast and primary lung cancer? Go all out Western medicine, or limit treatment to alternative modalities that align better with my spiritual sensibilities? As a practitioner of what philosopher Ken Wilber has called an "Integral Worldview" or metatheory, I was committed to do both at the same time. But how? I had taught the complexities of Integral theory over the years and knew that would be my orienting generalization.

Patricia recommended I read her disarmingly small book describing cell-level meditation. She explained her partnership with an extraordinary man, Barry Grundland, who practiced this healing modality. I am not a New Age advocate; I needed something that joined the ancient wisdom of the great minds with the most recent scientific findings.

Daily for several months, we worked together so that I could learn how to deeply touch my healthy and diseased cells in both my breast and lung. How, instead of "chomping them away" as many books described a Pac-Man approach to eating up the cancer cells, I was to teach the healthy cells to communicate with the diseased cells so they did not risk my life.

I've practiced many types of meditation over the years, but this was a level of depth I had never experienced. Slowly, I was able to contact my cells and began earnest discussions, teachings, directions. I was profoundly impressed when I learned that cells have an entire culture, society, containing my essence and my intelligence. I discovered I could breathe with and into the intelligence of the cells!

After both surgeries, which were fraught with complications, I was told I would have nine months of chemotherapy. Once again, I dug deeply into cell level meditation during that horrid period where all healthy and unhealthy growing cells were damaged.

I came through it all by November 2011, and Patricia had been my spirit guide, miracle healer. Until my oncologist told me about the metastatic lymph node...

I quietly sat down to meditate and affirmed that I must put my life into the hands of the healing techniques I had experienced by working with Patricia. For seven solid days I used cell level meditation with breaks only for meals and sleep.

I entered the operating room as my husband sat crying outside. I was draped so I couldn't see where the biopsy would be done on my left side. The room was cold; all were silent. The surgeon entered, and I could feel him use the ultrasound wand as he went up and down my left side above my shoulder. Minutes passed. Then I heard a whisper, "Get Dr. Smith from the OR next door." More minutes ticked away. Then I heard a swish of a door, and another doctor took hold of the wand. Back and forth he swept it. Finally, he removed the drape and said to me, "Go buy a lottery ticket. This must be your lucky day! That enlarged lymph node has completely disappeared!"

I bought the ticket. I didn't win. Instead, Patricia had once again helped me save my life.

Back to March, 2020. As I awaited the results of the test, I renewed my cell level meditation but this time a protective cocoon of crystal appeared around my body. I lay for hours in that state.

At midnight I was informed I did indeed have Covid-19, but with treatable symptoms, and I could return home in three days.

I am a litigating attorney, and I enjoy courtroom combat. I have a deeply spiritual side developed among several systems. I do not trust people easily and have never reached out for a "miracle cure." All I can affirm is that this beautiful, simple healing system has worked for me in the most difficult situations imaginable.

I owe my life to Patricia, and to cell level meditation.

Lynne D. Feldman, M.A., J.D.
Author of *Integral Healing*

Preface

Dr. Barry Grundland was a psychiatrist whose specialty area might have been called psychoneuroimmunology. This is a big word that basically means mind-body healing. The mind, including our thoughts, emotions and attitudes, affects the body, and in turn the body affects our minds, thoughts, emotions and attitudes. For over 50 years, Barry worked with people as a true healer—one who helps others come to Wholeness, or to a sense of being who they really are. Barry worked with people all over the world and helped them heal from things that modern-day medicine hasn't been able to cure.

He also worked creatively with some of the most evolved people on the planet to develop their talents more fully. He had a unique ability to meet people where they were developmentally or within their field of interest and to take delight in them. Of all his extraordinary accomplishments, he said he was most proud of his work and skills in child psychiatry.

It is Barry who named and developed the practice of Cell Level Meditation. He was never interested in writing, however. Once when I asked him about this, he replied that he didn't like to stop the flow of the Mystery. Somehow when we write about things, we define them, and Barry was more interested in experiencing the Mystery rather than defining it.

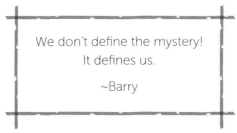

We don't define the mystery!
It defines us.

~Barry

In writing the "qualifications" that give me the authority to write this book, I confess first of all, I didn't go to medical school. One time, Barry said, "Thank God they didn't get their hands on you," which made me feel better for a while, but it is frankly something lacking in my development. Modern medicine is a treasure trove of very helpful information about our bodies! Perhaps Life meant me to develop in a deeply feminine, more organic way, since my true passions were more mystical, while wanting to be in service within the healing arts.

After college and a decade working in education, I moved to Mexico. My life shifted radically through childbirth. The experience was so powerful, I decided to become a midwife. When my son was two, our family moved back to the US, where I attended a very holistic midwifery school, in which I learned about such things as using creative visualization to help women connect with their bodies to get ready for labor and birth.

After my training was complete, we moved back to Mexico, where my husband (who was a doctor) and I founded a People's Clinic. The next decade I spent working as a midwife and learning about the life force through both birth and death; I had several near-death experiences during that time.

I also studied and worked with homeopathy, which is a unique study of the created order and a profound philosophy of healing! The last couple of decades brought me to live at the edge of a wetland, in the woods, where I have been privileged to go deeper into silence and to work with people as a spiritual director.

They say the teacher comes when the student is ready. I must say I've been blessed with many wonderful and generous teachers in my life. When I asked Barry if I could study with him by listening in on the sessions he would have with my husband when he got cancer, he was thoughtful for a while and seemed to be sensing into something. Finally, he said, "I'll work with you separately." And so, it began. Perhaps in the pause, the gods intervened. It was a fateful moment.

I had the privilege to work with Barry for over 15 years. There was an alchemy in our student/teacher relationship, which evolved over time. One day, he announced to me, "You're a colleague." Perhaps he knew I was ready to write the book, which came out of a living discourse between us over the years.

By writing it, we were ever mindful of the dangers of losing the very essence of an important quality of working within the Mystery: It is most alive when there is a dialogue going on and when relationship is being forged in the gap between one person and the other, and between the known and the unknowable. When someone asked Socrates why he never wrote anything, he said something like, "Wisdom happens in the space between two people in dialogue; it can't be written." It was his student Plato who wrote the dialogues he heard between Socrates and his students.

I wrote the book in a conversational tone, inviting you to engage an inner dialogue with your cells. Just start by talking with them. We'll give you some suggestions about what that conversation may be like and ways to enter into a deeper connection with yourself by meditating with your body. This is a book about experience and opening doors of perception to a deeper conversation with your embodied self.

Most of us learn to tune out or not attend to sensations in our bodies, so we may have to build the skills to rediscover this capacity to be aware of how intuition reveals information through sensations and feelings and memories and revelations in the body. By staying present for the experience, you add the breath. By staying present and open to your own experience: feeling, sensing, and finding the rhythm through the breath, things can change, all the way up and all the way down the ladder. Your gut relaxes and your anxiety lessens.

Your "older self" can reassure your "younger self" as you open doors of memory and deep feelings that are likely to emerge when you enter into meditative states for healing. One day, your younger self grows up and merges with your older self, in just the right way. By staying present, you notice how you are moved and by responding, breathing into and through your own experience, something comes to fullness, and wonder of wonder, something shifts! This shift can and does go all the way down to the way the cells are behaving, sometimes radically.

Barry thought people could become their own healers. Maybe. But, I tend to believe we need each other. You can find a friend, a healer, or a tree to engage in a dialogue, an interaction to allow yourself to be moved and changed and enlivened by something beyond your usual habits. Yet, we always have the breath, which is bigger than we are, so in a profound way, we are never doing this work "alone."

During the last few years of our relationship I became more of a confidant as Barry reflected on his own life and let me hear how things fit together in the whole from the altitude of age and wisdom. I listened and took notes. He spoke to me several times about letting go of all the "concepts" and going into the wilderness and having nothing. One day, he got very quiet and said, "Yes, I think you're ready. Let go of the concepts." He spoke about being totally naked and experiencing the Mystery and doing everything within this nakedness.

Not long after he stepped into this deep vulnerability, a young boy who had a rare brain disorder was sent to work with him. The boy was six years old and was pretty close to being a vegetable. On 23 Feb 2016,

Barry said, "I get the feeling that God is present and I'm with him in an almost hypnotic state. It's amazing how much love I feel for him. I'm focused on him as a child. Things come to me in that wonderful state I'm in. When I first met him, I thought, 'I don't know what to do.' I had to allow this feeling of inadequacy to be present. I feel vulnerable the whole time, and being vulnerable, I'm open."

By April, Barry told me: "I've seen God at work this whole time. I'm watching something occur that can only be God. He is beginning to walk and talk. He is infused with God because there's a radiance coming from him." Who would know that this would be the last "rational" conversation I would have with him, since Barry himself got some weird diagnosis within the following month and chose to go into hospice, since there was no known cure (he was 83).

He died 3 Nov. 2016. So, in retrospect we can see that this last great teaching was: a deeper surrender into "not knowing," and taking the last step into the Mystery, in which the gift of Love shows the way. Love is the way.

I am happy to republish this lovely book. I want Barry's work out in the world, whispering his words in people's ear.

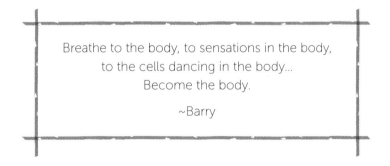

Breathe to the body, to sensations in the body,
to the cells dancing in the body...
Become the body.

~Barry

In other works on this topic I rarely see that last piece, where we are asked to become what is given to our awareness to observe. There is a pattern of observation, then interaction between subject and object (dialogue), then being moved by the interaction, and finally becoming and Being One with that which we are given to know. This finds its way into Wholeness in a way that is bigger than what we thought we knew. Barry was always and ever in surrender to the Mystery. And he was an incredibly curious and intelligent man who took great delight in the world and people and Life.

I have not changed much in this new edition of the book because there is a way in our modern lives that we want a blueprint that gets us stuck in our minds rather than entering into other ways of knowing where we can participate with something more lively in our natures. But I have added more stories and examples from people I've known. I worked to clarify the territory of the "Mind."

I have added more quotes from Barry, as I went back and reread his comments to me over the years. I added a chapter on Cell Level Theater to give an exercise that can help you enter into an experience of the cell through working with its functions. The book travels through our human sensibilities, naming them as something like "territories of awareness" so people can recognize them and engage them and move along into their own unique healing journey. I am giving you concepts. Once they are yours, you can let them go. It seems to happen in that order.

The Cell is a real thing in the material world, and it is a metaphor as well, since it carries a basic "pattern" of organization you can find at every level of Life. The cell has a nucleus, for example, which is a central area where you can find very basic information, that is very precise instructions for how things work; this information is inscribed on strands of tightly coiled threads called DNA.

In the Jewish Temple, there was a place called the Holy of Holies, where information for living holy lives that had been written on scrolls was kept. Only holy people, properly trained, could enter the Holy of Holies on certain prescribed days to read from the scrolls and take the information to the people. The solar system has a central sun that has a force which holds all the planets together and keeps them in order as they swirl through the Galaxy. The same pattern is revealed at different scales, no?

For our purposes, at the "level of the cell" we engage the workings going on there at different levels and states of awareness, which we can find with concentration, focus and participation through the breath. Barry was always leery of "defining the Mystery," but pointing in the direction of naming what is there and available to us as humans and just "average humans" at that, helps give people permission to go on their own journeys and to trust their own experience.

That's why I think he was happy with the book being written by the hand of a midwife, not a neuroscientist, although I can assure you, he loved neuroscientists as well.

Patricia Kay

The person who has all the questions
lives all the answers.

~Barry

Introduction

"May all things move and be moved in me
and know and be known in me.
May all creation dance for joy within me."

~Chinook Psalter
Quoted in: *A Grateful Heart*

Cell Level Meditation is a vehicle for finding our way "home." We take the breath to our cells, offering them our deepest desire to be happy and healthy and strong. In some way, they hear us and respond. (Or maybe we hear them asking for the breath!) This meditative form is a gift that helps the mind and the body come into healing, which in turn, helps us be ourselves in fullness.

In the Odyssey, the great mythological journey told by Homer, the hero, Odysseus, spends years trying to get home. To get there, he goes through all kinds of trials and tribulations. He must use every kind of skill and every clever device you can imagine. He always has to have his wits about him because something new and different is always coming up, and he has to have the courage of his creative response for each ordeal.

Of course, this is the archetypal human journey we all are on in one form or another. We are trying to find out who we are and how to be full in that. I would describe this as health: being fully who we are and having the body, mind and spirit in full congruence as an expression of that. As you begin taking this journey for yourself, you'll discover that the journey into the body, into the cells is quite an adventure! You can take it for your own creative reasons. This little book is a road map for the journey inside.

Many years ago, during a particularly difficult period in my life, I went to the beach in Mexico with some friends for renewal, healing and inspiration. One day, I was out swimming in the ocean, and as I was coming in, I got taken by a wave and was slammed against lava rocks at the shore's edge. I wasn't injured seriously, but my foot was scraped and bleeding. I was jarred by the experience of being taken by the powerful force of the ocean.

I stumbled out of the ocean with my scraped and bleeding foot. I was a little dazed, but I managed to walk down the beach where I sat under a huge rock. In the shade provided there, I intuitively went into deep meditation, experiencing fully the sensation in my foot without "doing" anything but noticing it and being present with the sensations.

Within seconds, an image came to me. In my mind's eye, I was seeing a moving kaleidoscope of orange shapes, like petals on a flower; the color was very brilliant. I was entranced by this spontaneous vision that came to me. I felt calmed by it. After a while in this meditative experience I began to "see" long, slender "fingers," purplish in color, coming together. I felt some excitement, and wondered if I were seeing Arnica flowers, since I'd never seen them. I am a homeopath, and certainly this is the remedy I would have taken if I'd had it with me, since Arnica is a plant used by herbalists and homeopaths to heal the trauma of bruised and injured tissue. I wondered if I were connecting with it, receiving its healing properties. By now, my foot no longer hurt, and I realized I had been healed. I opened my eyes and looked at my foot. The skin, which had been broken, was totally healed. There was only some minor redness left.

As you can imagine, I was amazed by this very dramatic healing. I felt touched by something very holy. I closed my eyes and went into this sense of amazement I was feeling. A question came to me: Did I want the power to heal people? I pondered this question and followed it down a path of self-inquiry. I discovered through this that I didn't want this power. From that clarification I also knew that what did (and does) interest me was accompanying people in their own discoveries of healing and unfolding and giving them any tools that might help them on their journeys.

I came out of my reverie and walked back down the beach to where my friends were. Now, one of the people I was with was my dear friend and mentor in homeopathy, Rosa. I asked Rosa what color Arnica flowers were, and she said, "They're orange." Then I wondered if I had connected with their essence in the first image given to me: the kaleidoscope of orange shapes. Because of the way my mind works, I believe I somehow captured what I call the "geometry" or the essence behind the form. And, I understood that the purplish "fingers" I'd seen were cells reuniting.

This was one of my more dramatic moments with Cell Level Meditation. It was about seven or eight months later that a friend told my husband and me to contact Barry, and we both began to work with him. Over the years of working with Barry, listening to him, and accompanying other people in their healing journeys, I have been blessed and delighted to travel into myself and others, to the cellular level and beyond. I have witnessed the ordinary power of the extraordinary bodies we live in as they (and we) come into healing, and I just love that!

Each cell is kind of a mini-world that contains the whole in a peculiar way. At the most basic of levels, each cell does all the things a whole body does: it breathes, it has intelligence, it takes in food and converts it to energy for creating new things, it cleanses itself, it renews itself and communicates with other cells. I also discovered that cells seem to have memories of events, beliefs, opinions, preferences, and habits. And there are color and movement, activity and rest, sounds and rhythm. They seem to be aspects of the template of life.

Sometimes as we are going into concentration to meditate with our bodies, we are given images, metaphors or clues to follow. These images are made for us, according to our own nature. Consciousness seems to get our attention in ways that are best meant for us. Some people don't get images at all, but rather they sense a rhythm or a tension or a stuckness that calls to them. We'll talk about this later. We are working with the notion of the analogue, in which a basic pattern reveals itself in different ways throughout different planes and states of awareness and manifestation. As I mentioned, the cell can be seen as the basic template for life and living systems.

I have also discovered that the inner journey inspires a similar kind of wonder and reverence as the outer journey. The journey in, or the journey out—they are surprisingly similar, and they seem to mirror each other. Looking out at the night sky inspires awe and reverence. We look up into the inky dark sky that holds glittery, sparkling lights and feel a deep sense of wonder. Going into the body—the tissues, the organs, the cells, the molecules and beyond—is similarly, breathtaking. The words spoken by the ancient master, Hermes Trismegistus ring true: "As above, so below. As within, so without." Yes! Wonder and reverence above and reverence and wonder below.

It's true, I was probably primed for the experience I described above. I began wondering about mystical things when I was very young. Then I learned to meditate just out of college. When I was in midwifery school in the 1980s, I learned about the power of guided visualization, through the work of Lewis Mehl-Madrona, Carl and Stephanie Simonton and Milton Erikson. In fact, I used guided visualization many times during my 12-year tenure as a midwife, sometimes with amazing results, and sometimes with disappointment. I had my doubts about it.

Being honest with doubt, looking it in the eye, acknowledging it's there and sometimes turning my back on it, helps me go to a deeper listening. Again and again, I am brought to a very humbling reality: healing is a mysterious journey. I don't control it. I don't get to decide who heals and who doesn't. I have a tendency to want to know the answers, to know how to do things, but again and again, this journey is about letting go into the moment with all my best instincts and letting the Mystery direct the unfolding.

It is much more beautiful and thorough than I am, and in fact, it's within the Mystery that healing happens.

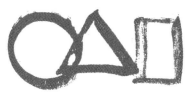

1

The Power of Meditation

"It is the mark of an educated mind
to be able to entertain a thought
without accepting it."

~Aristotle, philosopher
(384–322 BC)

Thanks to modern-day science, we've discovered that meditation can be a key factor in any healing program. Dr. Dean Ornish includes it in his program for cardiac patients. And, of course, Dr. O. Carl Simonton brought the experience of guided visual imagery to help people with cancer to heal back in the 1970s. Also, Dr. Bernie Siegel, along with many other medical doctors, were pioneers in showing the results of using guided imagery to bring healing to the body and its systems.

Dr. Mitchell Gaynor, an oncologist, has taught his patients to do a meditative chanting, which has been very healing for many of them. Joan Borysenko, Ph.D., clinical psychologist, co-founded and directed the Mind/Body Clinical Programs at the Beth Israel Deaconess Medical Center, Harvard Medical School. She has been one of the leading experts on stress, spirituality, and the mind/body connection in a universe which she says is "fundamentally mysterious."

Jon Kabat-Zinn, a professor at the University of Massachusetts Medical School, is well known for his work in mind-body medicine. He has found that patients trained in meditation have stronger immune systems than those who don't. And according to Ken Wilber, meditation training is the best way to accelerate the evolution of our consciousness. The Institute of Noetic Sciences (IONS), founded by the astronaut, Edgar Mitchell, is doing exciting research to bring Science and Spirit together, helping us to come to greater levels of understanding the reality of the mind-body connection.

These days, Mindfulness Meditation has become quite popular! There was a mindfulness study done in 2015 and in a retrospective analysis of about 4,500 people who completed a mindfulness integrative group intervention, 43% of those surveyed were less likely to need conventional medical services than their matched pairs!

In our culture, science is widely accepted as having the final say about what is "real." I get excited when Western science validates what has been described as a mystical experience by great thinkers through the ages. I get really excited when a structure I've "seen" in meditation within an organ or cell is revealed by a new imaging technology. Our culture believes in science, and it's important to us to have credible people doing well-designed studies to show us that we are doing something "real," not just indulging in wishful thinking. To help your scientific mind, I've listed a few resources at the end of this book so you can have a satisfying mind-experience of work that's been done to show that the mind-body connection is "real," and that meditation is effective. Each of these resources, in turn, directs you to many more resources. There is so much available these days to give you information and inspiration. All of these studies and books serve as compasses that point the way until you've had your own unshakeable experiences.

While respecting modern science, this book is not a science book. We are interested in exploring what happens when awareness is brought together with our living bodies, made of lively cells. The Quantum People (more science) tell us that when we look at something, we change it. The New Physics tells us that mind and matter are inseparably drawn to each other; they are mutually dependent! You can actually explore this for yourself. We want to tell you about experiences of our own and of other people we've known. Stories are powerful and open doors of possibility.

The perennial wisdom of great spiritual traditions has survived the test of time, while the "science" of every age up to now has been challenged, refined, and changed as our level of awareness and understanding has evolved. Maybe this just goes to show that our knowledge of the physical world isn't as "solid" as we might think. In fact, it may point to the notion that the very "solidness" of the physical world isn't as "real" or unchanging as we tend to think.

However, since recorded history, we have records of people pointing toward certain truths and spiritual principles that seem to hold up over time. These truths have a poetry about them. They quicken us when we hear or read them. They inspire us to our best selves. They lift us up. And they tend to show up in every tradition. The notion of treating others as we would like to be treated, known as the Golden Rule, for example, shows up in Christianity, Buddhism, Hinduism, Islam, and Judaism, just to name a few prominent spiritual traditions. And if you think about it and feel toward it, your body will sense the truth, the timeless truth of this statement, which we know as, "Do unto others as you would have them do unto you." It just feels right, no?

Yet, there has been a long-standing tension between Science and Spirit. David Ray Griffin, a modern philosopher and theologian summarizes the dilemma: "Whereas scientific beliefs are based primarily on sensory perceptions, religious beliefs are based primarily on non-sensory perceptions." The great religious leaders and great scientists have been trying to reconcile these differences for a long time.

Within this form of meditation, we may be evolving our capacity to deepen and expand our sensory perceptions, thus bringing science and spirit together in a fluid, interactive dance of greater understanding and reverence for the magnificent structures we live in: our bodies! Clear down at the level of the cells, we are healing the split, allowing each perspective its due, attending to our senses as well as staying open and in wonderment of things we don't know.

Master Nan Huai-Chi, a major source in the revival of modern Chinese Buddhism, made a startling statement that accords with this: "There's only one issue in the world: the reintegration between mind and matter." We live in a kind of illusion of a separate reality, where we dissociate. The ancient indigenous cultures knew that our existence is embodied sentience. The great spiritual traditions know this. It seems we "post-moderns" have to relearn this.

In our times, we continue to see the tension between the perspectives of science and spirit, the objective and subjective, the outer and the inner. I learned about Master Nan from listening to Peter Senge, who is a systems scientist at MIT! So, we are seeing a movement toward a more respectful relationship between science and spirit. Some of the research showing the connection between the mind and the inner or subjective self, and the body and the outer or objective self is very exciting (and comforting to folks whose intuition has been tuned this way). I must say, however, that while the studies help us and open us to exploration, they can also lure us into thinking that somehow, we can control what is deeply mysterious. I can hear Barry's words echo: "We don't define the Mystery! It defines us."

2

Cell Level Meditation in a Nutshell

"I wonder why. I wonder why.
I wonder why I wonder.
I wonder why I wonder why.
I wonder why I wonder."

~Richard P. Feynman, physicist
(1918–1988)

Let's begin to experiment with meditation. I am directing you toward three territories or places from which you can observe and participate.

1. The Silent Spaciousness

Notice the white part of this page…not the little black squiggles (the letters and words), but the white space.

This is no-thing-ness.

This is the background or the spaciousness the words are resting on. Notice what happens in your body when you just look at the white part of the page.

What do you notice?

Now, let's do something similar with the no-thing-ness all around you. There is a space around you where you know there is air. There is space between you and the ceiling. Right? Close your eyes and notice this space around you. Notice that there is spaciousness all around you. Take 30 seconds to do this.

What do you notice?

Perhaps you noticed that there is simply nothing there. Yes! That's right. There's nothing!

No-thing! How strange, no? Here we are noticing that there is no-thing-ness all around us. There's just empty space.

There is a place always around us in every moment where there is no-thing; where things aren't configured yet, where all possibilities lie.

There is silence. Just notice that there is silence, spaciousness, emptiness, no-thing-ness.

I don't want to put words in your mouth (or in your head), but if you really let yourself notice the space with nothing in it...

Could you sense something like peace, calm?

No-thing.

By noticing this silence, this empty spaciousness, just turning our attention toward it, we begin to open ourselves to new possibilities we hadn't thought to dream of.

We open ourselves to go beyond our programming. As you travel along this journey of cell level meditation, you will certainly be surprised again and again about how deep this programming is. Some of the programming is really great. Some of it is…well, less than really great. However, in the field of no-thing-ness, we can open up to things we didn't know to dream of, possibilities we never imagined. Oooh! The Mystery.

2. The Body

Very good! You have just had a very important experience in noticing silence and emptiness, no-thing. And that you can choose to notice it whenever you want.

Let's move on to the next step.

> Turn your awareness inward, to your body. Notice your body. There is definitely some-thing there, no? It's a substantial thing vs. the no-thing we were just noticing. There are lots of sensations you can readily identify. In fact, the body carries the "senses." There are many ways to approach the body. You can notice the whole body as one thing, part by part, tissues, bones, organs, and yes…cells.

One way to get started is to take a little trip through your body. I invite you to do this now, so you begin to cultivate some experience of your own. Starting with your head, let's explore the qualities of the body. See what sensations you can actually notice. Let your curiosity out and use all your senses to see what you actually notice. We'll go through each body part.

Beginning with the head: tune in and see what sensations you can be aware of in your head. Try to find a few words to describe anything you can notice (warmth, tingling, buzzing, heaviness, throbbing, and so on).

Move on down to your throat and neck. What can you detect there (tightness, openness, tension, green, purple, minty, bubbly, scratchy, sticky…)? Use all your senses.

Keep going down to your right arm—what do you notice?

Now, notice your left arm. Name the sensations you can detect there. You say nothing? How do you know it's there? Keep noticing.

Now, turn your awareness to your shoulders. What can you feel or sense there? Is there warmth, heat, pulsation, tightness, lead weight?

Keep going—what can you notice about your chest? Pay attention. What can you actually feel, sense or perceive in some way?

Maybe you are getting more relaxed and a vision will come to your mind's eye. It actually comes to you and you can notice it, so if that happens, it's there and you are beginning to tune into another plane of awareness.

Move down to the abdomen. What's going on there? Use your curiosity to see what you can actually notice and name (gurgling, rushing, green slime, hollow, a taste arising in your mouth, an odor).

The back? Notice vertebrae by vertebrae. See what sensations you can detect.

Go to your lower back, butt, hips and pelvis. What's going on there?

Now let's go down the left leg, all the way down to the knee, to the calf, to the ankle, to the foot. Get curious and see if you can be a good observer of what you can actually be aware of.

You're getting it: now go down the right leg: thigh, notice; knee, notice; calf, notice; ankle, notice; foot, notice.

Notice your feet on the ground, connecting to the earth. See what you can notice about that connection.

If my calculations are right, we've made it through the whole body, just noticing the sensations in each part. Do a quick body scan now and see if you can notice anything about the whole. Stop a minute and describe in words what you notice.

If you are like a lot of people I know, you may be surprised to discover how much you could notice just by turning your attention to your body's sensations. It's surprising how much is there, even on first glance, when you begin to pay attention. Remember my foot healing? This was all I did: notice. The foot healed itself.

3. The Breath

Ok, you now have an experience with no-thing and some-thing. Let's add one more thing:

The breath!

You are probably already breathing. Right? Now, I invite you to become aware of your breath:

Here I am
Breathing.
I breathe in.
I breathe out.
Here I am
Breathing in, Breathing out.
I feel the air coming into my nose.
I feel the air going out of my nose.
I feel the air coming in,

I notice the pause between breaths,
I feel the air going out,
I notice the pause.
I notice that without any thought at all,
The breath comes in, comes toward me.
From the silence, the breath comes toward me.
From the Great Space around me, the air comes into me.
I do nothing to cause this to happen.
The breath comes in, on its own.
I experience the rhythm of the breath
coming in and going out.
On its own, the breath of spaciousness comes in.
I breathe out and my breath goes to Spaciousness.
I feel wonder.
As I breathe out, I breathe into the wonder.
I breathe toward this sense of wonder.
I am filled with wonder.
I become this sense of wonder.
Wonder and I are the same thing!

But I get ahead of myself. Please take a little break and watch your breath. See what happens. What do you notice about paying attention to your breathing? Put this into a simple statement for yourself.

Let's go another step now. (You are moving along very quickly!)

You have noticed the spaciousness around yourself and no-thing, yes? You have noticed there are many sensations going on in your body. Maybe you noticed these sensations shifted a little just because you were noticing them. But, you have noticed some-thing.

You have noticed that you breathe in from the empty space around you. There is breathing going on.

Now, I suggest that you notice that you are breathing in from the space around you. For the first time, we are going to do something: direct the breath.

On the "out-breath," try taking the breath toward the sensations in your body. Pick one sensation that you can notice, and imagine that you are riding the breath into the body, bring it to the sensation. It's like blowing into a balloon. Fully breathe the breath toward the sensation, like sending a breeze in that direction. Notice.

Let the Great Space connect with the sensation on the wings of the breath.

Allow yourself to notice the sensation. Offer it the breath. See if you can breathe with that sensation. You and the sensation are breathing together, finding each other. Does the sensation seem to like the breath? Does it let it in? Can you go into the sensation with the breath?

Now Great Space, Breath and Sensation are one thing.

Open yourself to receive the breath from the spaciousness, breathe it toward the sensation. Take the breath up to the sensation. See how the sensation responds to the breath. Experience the sensation. Experience the breath and the sensation together. Pretend you are that sensation and see how the breath breathes. Experience breath and sensation in synchrony, breathing, shifting. Stay with it. Keep breathing…

What happened?

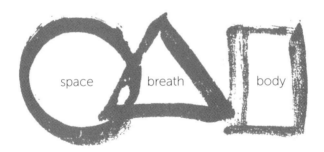

space   breath   body

There you have it. The ingredients of Cell Level Meditation are:

• Your awareness of the spaciousness around you or within you.

• Your awareness of the body and any sensations you have there, even if they are very subtle.

- From the spaciousness, breathe into your body, into the sensations you actually discover and become or merge with these sensations. (Keep going: noticing the next sensation, breathing into it, becoming it, and breathing as one.)

To Summarize

You might say that the one who is doing the noticing is "the mind" or awareness. The breath might be called "the spirit," and the body, is, well…the body! By paying attention, you bring these three aspects of yourself together.

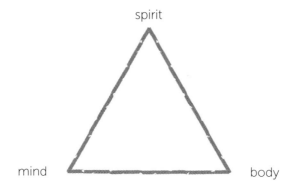

In the next three chapters, I'll explore each component of this triad a little more.

3

The Mind

"From the mind
Of a single, long vine,
One hundred opening lives."

~Chiyo-ni (1703–1775)

The Mind is the center of our intellect and understanding. What a gift it is to have a human mind which allows us to think, reason logically, consider options, learn language and math and science and history, morals and ethics and appreciate aesthetics. We can actually cultivate our understanding, knowledge, and appreciation of the world because we have minds. We can even consider and recognize whether something is True, Good and Beautiful.

When we study and commit ourselves to learning and applying understanding to our lives, we gain capacity, which in turn can lead to our experience of greater wonder and awe of this life we're given and the world we live in, not to mention our ability to participate and contribute.

When the Mind, which we usually think of as being "in the head" is connected to our hearts (what we care about) and to our bodies (our instruments of perception and action), we are actually in harmony with and aligned with ourselves in very beautiful ways. When the Mind is not connected, there can be serious problems.

The Mind thinks thoughts. That's what it does. Unfortunately, if we're only paying attention to our thoughts, we can be disconnected from our bodies, from our feelings, from our priorities, from what we really care about. From what we love. This is a problem because we get disconnected from our natural Wholeness.

In this chapter, I want to point toward this little problem so you can recognize when it's happening to you, and so you have a tool to work with it. Basically, the Mind can move out of the moment, and lose its guiding purpose, and its connection with the body. It can get lost in aimless, distracted free-association or "thought-thinking." In fact, we're going to name this rascal, "the disconnected thought-thinking mind," so we can talk about it.

We can be "over mentalized" these days. We can be "all in our heads," thinking thoughts with no skin in the game. It's not uncommon to get lost in this random "disconnected thought-thinking" when we meditate, in a way that actually keeps us from going into deeper states of awareness.

Several years ago, a friend came over to visit. I was in a state of despair. After listening to me, all she said was, "Wow, you're really in your head!" She was right, and I felt her love and insight crash through the darkness where my "mind" knew all the answers to everything and was making me miserable! My mind was like a "Talking Head," disconnected from the moment, from my body, from the beauty around me, and my friend's sweet presence.

So, we want to be wary of a "disconnected-thought-thinking" that can take over and keep us from connecting to and aligning with ourselves more deeply. The "Talking Head" is not present in the moment, it may be wandering around in the past or wondering about the future, analyzing a situation without heart or concern. There is often a random quality to it—thoughts ramble around without focus, going in loops that lead nowhere and for no good purpose. There can also be a frantic quality to it because it's lonely and untethered from anything greater than itself.

Let's make a slight distinction which will be useful later. Let's distinguish between Mind and Awareness. Our minds think thoughts. Our Awareness is broader, it simply notices. In fact, Awareness can notice: "I'm thinking thoughts."

Awareness is a little like the Sky. The clear blue sky. It is open and vast. The mind is like a cloud that is very beautiful, and it moves through the clear blue sky. Neither one is right nor wrong, rather they are just features of our human experience. We have awareness and we have minds.

Here is a little experiment:

- Just notice, for a moment, that something in you is Aware. (This is a major miracle by the way.)

- Something in you is reading along, following the words on the page.

- If you were to ask Awareness to look away from the page, who does that?

Perhaps you have just noticed that
something in you is aware,
and
something in you can "direct awareness"
or choose where you place your attention!

Astonishing, no?

We want to notice: we have awareness.

Something in us can stand back and bear witness,

to detect a movement or a sensation arising,

a thought coming along.

In fact, we want to notice that we notice.

Something in us notices there are clouds in the sky,

moving in and out of different patterns.

We didn't make the sky or the clouds,

but there they are!

Awareness is such a wonderful thing to have.

Choosing where to focus awareness connects us to ourselves.

Sky or Clouds?

We want to acknowledge that Awareness holds the Mind,

But goes beyond the Mind.

Awareness is the capacity to notice whether and that you're noticing. And, Awareness itself can be developed into exquisite forms of self-reflection that can give you more freedom and appreciation of life. It can even help you meditate and engage your cells!

Learning to notice the quality of awareness itself is very practical. Whoa! Awareness can be aware of Awareness! If you step back a moment, you can discern whether your awareness is:

Open,

    Bored,

        Focused,

    Suspicious,

      Timid,

        BOLD,

    Snarky,

Humble,

      Certain,

    Uncertain,

        Cynical,

     Fearful,

       Foggy,

Sleepy,

    Precise.

Just to name a few qualities we all have experienced. The quality of your awareness hugely influences what you are able to notice! For example, if you're closed down, not much information can come to you. If you are open, more information can come to you. If you are too open (unfocused), you can be overwhelmed. So, noticing the quality of your awareness is very practical, no?

For our purposes, we acknowledge that we have Awareness which is noticing things. The quality of awareness is a filter which determines what we can perceive. We want to develop the capacity, over time, to notice the quality of our awareness. Awareness can develop a lovely receptivity to higher kinds of information beyond our categories, when we're ready.

We want Awareness to be alert, to notice when "disconnected-thought-thinking" has taken over. Ah...I see you are "thinking thoughts" and that you have separated from the moment, from the body, and in fact, from what really matters to you! Rather than scold the "disconnected-thought-thinker," Awareness can direct the "thought-thinker" to assess whether it's connected with the body, with what's good, with a clear goal.

Once the thought-thinker has a clear job, it's happy! It can discern if you're connected to what you care about. It can make your meditation more precise, by asking: where are the cancer cells? It can keep you focused on your intention. Your thought-thinking mind loves being helpful and helping you connect to a higher purpose. When it does this, you can be rescued from endless loops that get stale and tiresome and rob you of your life energy. When Awareness has detected that the disconnected-thought-thinking mind has taken over, you can direct it to focus on the goal or to articulate an important question.

A very useful practice when you sit down to Meditate with your cells, is to find an intention to give focus, which will ground your meditation. I love the word "intention." It's strange to love a word, but words are so powerful and can help us be both precise and connected to the source of a tradition from which they come. In this case, "intention" comes from the Latin word, "intentio," which means aim, purpose, aspiration. I think of it as "tending" toward something. What am I tending toward that brings greater coherence, aim and purpose to order my life? You may be amused to learn, as I was, that "distraction" comes from the Latin "distrahere," which means: to drag apart or to pull in a different direction. We want the power of focused intention, bringing our body, mind and spirit together.

Take a few minutes to discover what purpose or aim you're "tending toward" as you begin your meditation. You have to go beyond "thought-thinking" to discover this. So, try getting quiet, and turn toward the spacious silence. The Sky. Allow Awareness to rest in the place beyond thoughts. Just empty spaciousness. Just sweet silence. From that sweet silence, notice that the silence and you are breathing together. Take a moment to be present with your breath. Feel your whole body breathing, the rhythm, the in, and the out.

Let your Mind ask a good question: "What do I need from this meditation so I can heal?" "What do I really care about?"

Then let go, be still and be open to what comes to you. The answer may come as a word, a phrase, a gesture, an image, a symbol, or an intuition. Be open and see what comes to you out of the Silence, however it comes to you. When it comes, check it out with your body. Your body knows when things are true, and so, when you sense into an intention and give it a name as the goal for your meditation session, your whole body will "tend toward" that. Your Cell Collection will say, "yes." You'll feel it! When the mind and the body are in congruence there is a sense that feels right. You feel at ease. How interesting that when there isn't congruence, you experience the opposite: dis-ease.

Can you see and feel that the thought-thinking mind is not inventing the intention, but rather discovering what's really true from a deeper, more connected source? Once this discovery is made the thought-thinking mind can frame the intention as a statement that will help you focus, like a mantra which calls you back to your intention. It finds and chants the right word or phrase to keep you focused. If you shine a flashlight on an object in the dark, that is where your attention goes, no? The spiritual teachers have a catchy phrase that goes: "Energy flows where attention goes."

Your focused intention is the flashlight. Once you have connected to it, you will have a powerful aid in helping you open up to the places in yourself, your body and your cells that may need a better "arrangement."

One time, I told Barry about an amazing discovery a woman I was working with had made in a session with me. As he listened, he said, "She lost her focus; that has nothing to do with her healing." It was true! She got side-tracked! She was seduced by a flashy distraction (and I was too). In retrospect, I think Barry could feel the disconnection! Sometimes, you learn to say "no," and return to your intention, which has come to you and serves you.

When your intention has come to you out of the Silent Spaciousness, let go and begin to notice your breath. Connect with the experience of breathing. Allow your body to guide you by noticing sensations, images or sounds that you can perceive. Stay alert! Stay present to all the sensations as they come to you, and notice where you're drawn. As you go toward that, you are bringing along your care, curiosity and the breath. This is your offering. As you are opening, being guided toward sensations that call for the breath, and breathing with the sensations, your state of consciousness (the quality of your awareness) may change. Your brainwaves will probably be shifting into a coordinated rhythm that allows you to be more present in your experience and to find the pattern of healing that is most useful in that moment or meditation session. You may have a heightened sense of awareness. You may notice a kind of liveliness that you hadn't really seen before—a liveliness that's always there and strangely familiar. However, it's different now, because your state of awareness is connecting you to it in a new way.

There are many ways this may happen for you, and I feel compelled to tell you so that you can stay open and not get stuck in the idea you're doing it wrong. Everyone has different proclivities, and you'll discover this all the way down to the cells. Some people are very visual, and they tend to "see" things in their "mind's eye." Other people "hear" things; they hear a tone or a hum and have a sense of whether they experience harmony or dissonance, whether it "feels right to them" or not. Others have a kind of epiphany, and suddenly, they just know things; it's hard to describe how they know them, but their bodies are enlivened and re-ordering from this revelation. I knew a woman who would go into a cold sweat and shiver when this happened to her, as if her whole body were being rearranged.

Stay present for whatever comes your way. Bring the breath to travel into the sensations and stay present with them. Stay exquisitely present with your experience, second by second, breath by breath. There is great power in staying present even with difficult things. These very difficult things often have in them the seeds of just what you need for healing. You will discover this in your own time, but I'm whispering in your ear now, so you stay present and focused with your true heart's desire.

But, we're not thinking about these difficult things, we are experiencing them as wisdom in our bodies and breathing with them. What's happening at the cell level is already happening. Go into it. Be with it. Be curious about it and bring the breath to it and then join in and breathe with it, just as it is. You may feel a tingling somewhere in your body—stay present to it as an experience. Breathe with that experience. If you are working on your liver, see how it calls you. Maybe you'll sense a slight pressure under your ribs.

Once you are curious about the sense, you allow yourself to experience that sense. You bring along the breath, your offering from the Great Space, and breathe into and with the sense. Notice how your liver responds. If a color shows up in your mind's eye, experience its effect on you, how it might move you, how it affects the quality of your awareness. Join in and breathe along with it. Keep going. Stay present in the experience; the thought-thinking mind can analyze it later and draw conclusions. In fact, the thought-thinking mind can give words for you to write in your journal after the meditation is over, so you can track your progress.

Life speaks to us in such wonderful ways! And by Minding your Mind with focus, choice, and care, Mind and Matter come together, joined by the breath of Being in the body. You may just have a healing.

I worked with a 7 year-old boy
who had Crohn's Disease; it was genetic.

He was going to have a resection
of his colon. He was on cortisone.

I said to him:

"Here's what I'd like you to do
and think about:

What do you do to rebuild
the intestine?"

After 12 sessions,
he said to his parents:

"I'm done, cured."

He went in there
and became the disease.

~Barry

4

The Body

"The great wisdom dwells in the body.
Fully away from all thoughts, it dwells in the body,
but is not produced in the body."

~A Sambhuti (Buddhist) text

I must say, the human body is quite a wonder. It is a very brilliant organism, made up of living cells. The cells are actually alive and responsive. They are the smallest living units. They are quite amazing. And they get together, in communities, and make up tissues and organs. These get together and give rise to the whole body. Trillions of cells get together, get along, and orchestrate life through the body.

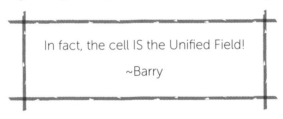

In fact, the cell IS the Unified Field!

~Barry

The capacity of the body to stay healthy most of the time and to bring about its own healing from all kinds of disorders is quite amazing. Sometimes, it becomes even more intelligent by getting well from an illness as if something comes to greater awareness or a higher level of functioning as a result.

"...I may have been beaten down by cancer, but I did rise—taller, stronger, more vibrantly alive than before."

—Ruth Ann McCann, alumna of a cancer retreat
at Harmony Hill in Union, Washington

Another woman echoes these words:

"A part of me died. It had to happen, so something new could be born. I never thought I'd say this, but I am actually grateful for the cancer. I never would have come this alive had I not come through this journey. Now, I'm in partnership with all these different dimensions of me."

—Debbie Hansen

What startling statements! Actually, not uncommon from people who have healed from terrible diseases. By engaging the body consciously, you can discover all kinds of things about yourself.

And, after having sung its praises, I will also state that the body is quite a taskmaster! When it's out of order, you're miserable! Now this body of ours, as you already know, is made up of basic building blocks—cells. Each cell is a little world that is quite lively.

Surrounding each cell is an outer covering, the cell membrane, which has a great intelligence about what is allowed in and out of the cell. This membrane has channels in and out of the cell, receptor sites that allow it to receive messages from other parts of the body. It makes decisions about who gets in and who stays out. Inside of the cells, all the functions are going on that keep the whole body alive: breathing, drinking, eating, eliminating, consuming and producing energy, reproducing, communicating, and being creative. And, you may be surprised to learn that the cell is responsive—it seems to enjoy attention. In fact, it seems to enjoy the same things you do!

Candace Pert, Ph.D., was a research professor in the Dept. of Physiology and Biophysics at Georgetown University Medical Center in Washington, D.C. Her descriptions of the biological capacities of cells are striking. She discovered that there is dynamism involved between thoughts and cell responsiveness. The "stuff" of our bodies is not just inert and inanimate, but rather it is constantly shifting, changing, responding to conscious and unconscious signals. She also noticed that the body actually responds to what we think, and we probably are responding to what it thinks as well. She wrote:

> "Emotions and bodily sensations are intricately intertwined in a bi-directional network in which each can alter the other. Usually this process takes place at an unconscious level, but it can also surface into consciousness under certain conditions or be brought into consciousness by intention."

Furthermore:

> "There are almost infinite pathways for the conscious mind to access—and modify—the unconscious mind and the body."

This is a powerful statement—almost infinite pathways!

Practically unlimited possibilities! The actual physical structures that are created in the cell as the dialogue between mind and body is going on, is an exciting area of discovery, showing us that our thoughts are literally creative of such things as new polypeptides, hormones, new neural pathways and things way beyond the scope of this book.

When you start to explore this vast intelligence of matter itself, as it lives in your physical body, you will discover yourself, again and again.

The imprint of who you are is in every cell. As Jon Kabat-Zinn would say, "Wherever I go, there I am."

Once I worked with a woman during her pregnancy.

By the ninth month, her baby had not yet "descended" into the pelvis, which is something that happens in the last month of pregnancy for most women. The baby's head flexes as she or he puts the chin down on the chest, allowing the dimensions of the head to fit into the mother's pelvis in the right way for birth.

This woman was very good with meditation. Every day, she entered into contact with her baby and told her, "Put your chin down. Put your chin down."

Sure enough, the last week of pregnancy came and the baby's head descended into the correct position in her mother's pelvis. The birth went fine, although it turned out the baby had a large head!

When this young child was about 2 and just learning to talk, she turned to her mother one day and said, "Put your chin down! Put your chin down! Right, Mamá?"

~Patricia

5

The Breath

"The sky gave me its heart
Because it knew mine was not large enough to care
For the earth the way it did."

~Rabia of Basra, Muslim Sufi Saint
(717–801 AD)

The breath, the simple act of breathing, is the cornerstone of many types of meditation. In many languages the words for breath and spirit are the same. You might contemplate the breath and the act of taking in air, the sensations you experience as you do this, the fact that you do it without thinking about it, the fact that the air is always there for you, the fact that it's free and it's freeing. There is something quite uplifting, expansive and wonder-evoking just in the simple act of breathing. And I've heard that every breath is unique! Like a snowflake!

The breath is associated with the spirit. To get a sense of this we can ask, what does it mean to do something "in the right spirit?" When you do something in the "spirit" of generosity, for example, how do you feel? If you do something in the spirit of vengeance, how do you feel? By considering "the spirit" with which we are engaging life, we are exploring another aspect of the "quality of awareness." In the Justice System, we talk about the "letter of the law" as compared to "the spirit of the law." When the "letter of the law" becomes too rigid, it can kill the original intent of goodness the law was meant to protect, right?

Of course, this points to deep ethical questions that have complexity and challenge us to grow…in spirit…to get in touch with what we really care about. People who commit crimes and find themselves in jail often come to regret having done something they knew was wrong and they talk about their "lower passions" getting the better of them: greed, envy, pride, lust, vanity, hatred. There seems to be something in most people that really does want "the good."

I knew a detective who told me he noticed that people have a deep yearning for their lives to be "made right," and so they often leave some clue that will lead to their getting caught. So, reaching to the "sky," the Great Space for a "spirit of goodness" beyond our small-mindedness and lower passions has great potential to uplift us to something greater than we knew to hope for. Your part in this is to let Awareness open you to something greater, something where your own spirit is made right. You can open to hope rather than despair, to kindness rather than meanness and then … the Sky is the Limit, you lift your heart to the Great Space and participate with the breath. You breathe.

Each time you breathe, you are participating in the Mystery! When you do this with some awareness, you may have an experience of awe and wonder. The Vastness of the Infinite comes into the finite body. The Spirit connects the Heaven with the Earth – it is the link between them! With awareness, you can take in the breath and follow it into your earth-place, your very body. This Great Space which is around the whole earth, is so big, and it comes into your nose, down your throat, into your trachea, into your lungs, down, down, down into increasingly smaller and smaller passages, all the way into these delicate sacks, like tiny balloons, called alveoli in the lungs. The surface of the alveoli is only one cell thick. The Mighty Breath has now come down to this delicate membrane and crosses over into the one-cell-thickness of a capillary (smallest blood vessel) to be received by the blood cells, which in turn will travel all through your body to deliver the Mighty Breath to every single cell. The Great Space makes itself very small, very refined, very calibrated to your exact needs. Whoa! I find this mind-boggling!

And for our purposes, and this is very important, the Breath opens the channels of healing. The Breath takes us beyond the thinking of the disconnected-thought-thinking, problem-solving small mind (that it is in charge of healing). The Breath opens the body and the mind to infinite possibilities.

It connects us to no-thing-ness, beyond our conditioning, our programming and our habits, to possibilities not yet dreamed of. It stops us from "thinking" we are doing the healing and opens us to The Great Healing. What a relief!

Stillness: we have to come to it; it's the step to the Knowing.

In the Knowing, we go to the Unknowing.
At that point, it's all energy.

By using focused intention and breathing, you have set up in the body a communication that was never there.

You cannot fail in this process; if you stop breathing you die.

~Barry

Breath!
Great Spirit!
Here I am!
From the Great Space, I breathe.
I breathe into this body.
The Spirit moves over the form of the earth—
My body, this piece of earth.
I open to this Great Spirit,
Breathing.
In and out.
With the Great Spirit,
I breathe into this body.

I open to where the Breath leads.
I experience the rhythm of the breath.
I experience the sensations that meet the breath.
I become those sensations and see how the breath breathes
Into them,
With them,
Through them.

We are breathing together this Great Breath and me.
Where there is a color, the breath shifts, and we breathe.
Where there is a hum, the breath tunes in, and we breathe.
Where there is movement and rhythm, the breath dances,
and we breathe.
Where there is tightness, the breath slows down, and we breathe.
Where there is openness, the breath gets bigger, and we breathe.
So many ways to breathe with the Spirit
Moving over the waters of my Being
Calling my Cells into harmony with
My True Heart's desire.
Breath into the very cells of this human body
Dancing their way into my life.
Here I am!
Already Whole,
Here I am!

6

Not Knowing & Knowing Too Much

"A hidden connection is stronger than an apparent one."

~Heraclites, philosopher
(535–475 BC)

We only have fragments from this Greek philosopher, but this statement is one of those perennial truths that's been on record since around 500 BC. Another angle on this, expressed in modern times:

"Every event has in it the nature of a surprise, a miracle or something you could not figure out."

~JR Oppenheimer, nuclear physicist
(1904–1967)

When you begin to meditate, you don't know what will come toward you. You don't have to know. In fact, it's probably what you don't know that has the greatest power and holds the greatest potential for your true healing. Remember the analogy of shining the flashlight in the dark room? Your intention shines that flashlight, but what steps into the beam of light, coming out of the darkness, is often quite a big surprise.

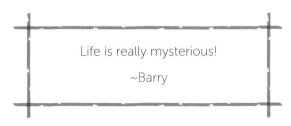

Life is really mysterious!

~Barry

Being able to stay open to "not having to know everything" is such a liberating gift. Don't worry, though, your mind will probably pop up over and over, trying to take charge, asking things like, "Why?" Many people I've worked with have done a lot of therapy and have all kinds of insights into their past. This is good. One thing that can get in the way, however, is jumping too quickly to a decision, "Oh, I've already seen this, and this is why this is happening to me."

One woman who worked with me came up with a great line to help herself when she noticed this happening: "Uh, oh! The 'whys' got me again." And then she'd go back to the silence, the experience of the body and the breath. And remember, you can help your mind stay curious by helping it ask better questions, like, "Where is that going on in the body?"

Sometimes you think you're going to heal something. You begin to breathe, and the breath takes you down a totally unexpected trail, opening doors, liberating cramped and musty ideas for a deeper healing in body and mind than you ever thought possible. Or, continuing with the flashlight analogy, monsters, vampires, and three-year-olds with sad faces step into the spotlight. You just never know what's going to show up. This can be a little scary!

Elephant Wondering

A seed
Has sprouted beneath a gold leaf
In a dark forest.

This seed is seriously contemplating,
Seriously wondering about
The moseying habits
Of the Elephant.

Why?

Because
In this lucid, wine-drenched tale
The Elephant is really –
God,

Who has His big foot upon us,
Upon the golden leaf under which lies
This sprouting
Universe

Wherein
We are all a little concerned
And

Nervous.

~Hafiz, Sufi poet and mystic
(1313–1390)

It seems strange to say that there are some dangers that go along with knowing too much. I realize it's not that I do, in fact, know too much, I just think I know too much. The great sages would point out that you can't put more water in a glass that's full. Somehow, when I "think I know," I'm not able to be receptive and open. I'm not available for something new or different or more nuanced to come to me because my "know-it-all" self has closed the door. I'm certainly not as alert or curious, and I don't seem to get as far or as deep in my meditations.

"In the beginner's mind there are many possibilities, but in the expert's there are few."

~Shunryu Suzuki, Zen Buddhist monk
(1904–1971)

Because of the experiences I've had of being surprised and delighted when this quality of "know-it-all" has gotten out of the way, I have been able to cultivate more trust that what needs to come forth will. This is true for me if I am meditating on my own or with another person. In fact, over the years, I have come to trust the "I don't know" place as a doorway into the unsuspected breakthrough, a miracle waiting to happen! Don't worry! We still have our rootedness in what we "know as good." We are not throwing everything out, but we are being open to something even more wonderful coming forth.

We often speak of people who have this irritating habit, as "close-minded," no? In my case I have had to temper certain kinds of "objective," "scientific" information with a sense of wonder and awe about the incredible capabilities of the body. I have witnessed these capabilities, which often seem miraculous. Bring science and mystery together with…you guessed it! The Breath!

The moon rises slowly over the pond, peeking out above the trees.
I read somewhere that the moon is 238,855 miles from the earth.

Oh! This luminous wonder stops me in my tracks
and holds me in its gaze.
I read somewhere that the moon is made of
a rocky silicate composition.

The moon is a numinous presence; oh, look!
This round wonder smiles down from on high.
I read somewhere that the moon has a surface gravity
about one-sixth that of the Earth.

Oh, Moon! The kids and I chant with glee,
"I see the moon and the moon sees me.
God bless the moon and God bless me!"
I read somewhere that the gravitational influence of the moon
produces the tides of the Earth.

Dear Moon, Powerful Mover of the Tides! You follow along from
the sky with me on the ground, lifting my thoughts
to awe, to beauty.

I do like the material facts, and I would certainly want them if I
were going to build a rocket ship.

But, they don't take my breath away
In quite the same way.

I read somewhere that when the first men went to the moon
in their rocket ship,
They turned back and beheld: the Earth rising ~
And they were overcome by awe.

So, cultivate "not knowing" and childlike curiosity—simply wonder—
and let the softness of your gaze open up. Don't ruin the Mystery!
And—be prepared for delightful surprises!

Having said this, understanding the "mechanics" of how something
works can also be quite exhilarating. Biologists and quantum physi-
cists are discovering all kinds of new information. We have imaging
technologies that are confirming our inner "seeings." If you study a
medical text about what's going on physiologically, it may open you to
see things you wouldn't notice if the idea, image or concept hadn't been
stimulated into your awareness by being exposed to it in a book. If you
have diabetes, for example, studying all the dynamics of the pancreas,
the production of insulin, and the responsiveness of the cells to glucose
is a great idea.

Just keep in mind that our bodies are amazing organisms that work
with incredible intelligence, so we want to be cautious about limiting
their creative and curative responses by our limited understanding of
how they work to begin with.

One time, I showed a film on the body (down to the cell level) to
an on-going Cell Level Meditation class I was leading. One man was
working on healing a bone that had fractured and wasn't healing properly. He'd had a stunning breakthrough one week! He saw color, energy,

movement and was really able to get in with the healing breath. His pain level was minimal when he left that evening. It was the following week when I showed the film. Then we did the meditation and he was so disappointed! He told me I'd ruined it for him. What was true and powerful and healing for him had come to him spontaneously, in a way that was meant for him. We each find our own way.

I am reminded of Bruce Lipton's story of being ostracized by his colleagues when he discovered that the cell membrane has intelligence. In fact, he considers it the "brain" of the cell, instead of the nucleus! Bruce Lipton is a cell biologist who has discovered many of the things this book is about in the laboratory. However, when he tried to share this with his colleagues, the information threatened their world view of how they thought things worked, and so they couldn't accept what he was showing them. Yet…

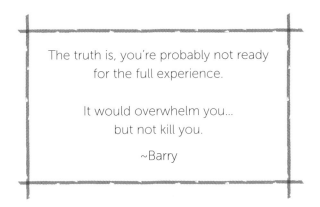

The truth is, you're probably not ready
for the full experience.

It would overwhelm you...
but not kill you.

~Barry

7

Falling? Dive!

"And so accept everything which happens, even if it seems disagreeable, because it leads to this, the health of the universe…For [Zeus] would not have brought on any man what he has brought, if it were not useful for the whole."

~Marcus Aurelius, Roman Emperor
(121–180 AD)

Whatever comes toward you as you take this journey inside your body, you can dive in. Once I talked to a guy who liked to climb rocks. He told me something very amazing. He said that one time when he was climbing, he fell. For a brief moment he experienced fear, and then he moved beyond the fear and decided to go into the fall as if he were diving. And, he managed to land on the ground in a way that he didn't even get hurt.

Cell Level Meditation can be like this. Instead of recoiling in fear or helplessness, you may choose to jump into whatever comes toward you. Ride the breath into it. Notice the sensation/color/sound/smell; experience it; take the breath into it; become one with it and breathe some more. Keep going!

So, breathe into your body with curiosity. Ride on the breath toward the cells. Dive into whatever comes toward you. Trying to fix it and don't know what to do? Notice where that thought lives in your body (maybe tightness in your shoulders or clenching in your jaw), then breathe into the "trying to fix it"! Fully experience the sensation and breathe! If a sad cell comes toward you…hmm…what is your response? Can you allow your body the experience of sorrow or do you need to tell it to "get a grip and keep going?" All the way inside, you find out who you are. And there's only one you in all the world. Use your own creative response to whatever is your true experience. And breathe to it!

If an evil cell comes toward you…hmm…what will you do? Now you may have to engage in such philosophical questions. And the cells and the breath may reveal some surprises that inform your life in interesting ways. I can tell you that wherever I have encountered evil, there has been a profound disconnect…like a disembodied mind that was not aware of its interconnectedness and interdependence with others. So, if you deal with cells that have no interest in being in relationship with other cells, you may need to restrain them and help the body activate ways to keep them from hurting the others, including moving them right on out of the body, or retraining them to be helpful (like the bacteria in the gut that helps digest your food, but is not allowed to get in the blood and wreak havoc). How you deal with such a deep question reveals the depths and proclivities of your own nature, your own special genius, as well as a way you are learning from, adapting to and adjusting through your own experience.

It often happens that you begin Cell Level Meditation with the desire to heal something wrong with your physical health, but by breathing into what is given to you, fully experiencing what comes to you, you end up finding out who you really are and what you're good at or what's really important to you. Perhaps, this is how heaven and earth come together: the Spirit (the breath) comes in to animate your embodiment as a human (earth). This is the true healing. And! Our bodies don't lie, so listen watchfully! Take the breath to the place, quality, or sensation the body points toward, and dive in there.

Now I will give you a little preview that you may find tantalizing.

Consider: The Stem Cell!

A few years ago, in experiments with mice, researchers showed that they could wipe out a cell's developmental "memory" by inserting just four genes. Once returned to its pristine, embryonic state, the cell could then be coaxed to become an altogether different type of cell.

In 2010, scientists built on this work with spectacular results. Two research teams took cells from patients suffering from a variety of diseases and reprogrammed them into stem cells.

The transformed cells grow and divide in the laboratory, unlike most adult cells, which don't survive in culture conditions. The cells could then be induced to assume new identities, including those cell types most affected by the diseases afflicting the patients who had donated the initial cells.

This was done "mechanically," what if we reprogram the cells via … awareness plus breath?

> Each cell is the same as every other cell. Then it changes and becomes whatever specialized cell is needed by the body.
>
> ~Barry

Each type of cell in the body has its own characteristics, but it also holds a certain basic and profound similarity with all cells. You may discover that bone cells have a different "feel" to them than, let's say, nerve cells. Bone cells have a different function than nerve cells. They are keeping the structure together, while nerve cells are carrying information all through the system, delivering messages from Headquarters. Now, "holding structure" can be quite vibrant. Subjectively, these two functions feel different.

Just notice how you experience things as they are, taking the breath to them, becoming them, "matching" your breath to the sensations. You may find it useful to notice the speed or frequency at which something is expressing itself. Then, slow down or speed up to "match" the speed so you can join in. Breathe slower, wait, allow, let awareness shift to meet what comes forth.

Perhaps you are more tuned into sound. Some people hear tones and humming when they go into their bodies. So, if you hear a tune, try matching your voice to it, just like listening to the concert master, who sounds the note on which everyone should start to sing. Listen for the note and match your breath to it. Become one with it.

I'll give you an example. Once I tripped over a log and fell down flat, face down. Immediately, I met the whole sensation exactly as it was, using my voice out loud. I stayed with this sensation for several minutes, using my breath/voice. Now, if you think about having such a startling accident, you can imagine the noise that came out of me was intense and almost primal, like an animal howling.

It seems that by meeting my true experience of the situation in this way, within minutes the pain and shock were gone. I got up and there was never any bruising, no after-effect of swelling, soreness, or stiffness. Healing came about instantly. And if you think about it, perhaps this is why we spontaneously cry out, "Ouch!" when we hurt ourselves—it's a form of cell meditation! The point is, if you experience something intense in your body, meet it with something equally intense. Instead of trying to calm yourself down, meet the intensity of what is happening, as it is happening.

Go into it with curiosity; simply wonder. Become it and breathe, taking spaciousness into the center of it all. Things rearrange and transform when they're ready!

Barry told me about a young boy he was working with by having him draw the progression of his healing.

One day, he told me he really had to resist the temptation to direct the boy.

"I have 50 drawings. I keep wanting him to get to the kidneys, but I restrain myself. He's not quite there yet."

Barry was a master at meeting people right where they were with exquisite restraint and curiosity.

8

Emotions

"Why look you,
how you storm!
I would be friends with you and have your love."

~William Shakespeare, playwright
(1564–1616)

Sometimes, when you're traveling around in your body, you might come upon an emotional feeling. Of course, you know that the sensation you have inside when you're angry is different than when you're sad, which is different from loneliness or from excitement. It is tempting to go into thoughts about the emotion (why you think it is there).

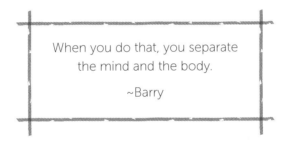

When you do that, you separate
the mind and the body.

~Barry

Try noticing the sensations in the body that the emotion evokes. That's where you go in. Experience the sensation in the body, evoked by the emotion. Match your breath to the sensation and let Mystery do the rest. Perhaps a deeper healing is at hand. Breathe and breathe some more. Let the breath do the work!

Sometimes when you go into a meditative process engaging the cells, you may find yourself steeped in memories that evoke strong emotions. The cells seem to store our life histories, and I believe, the life histories of our ancestors. Because the larger intelligence of the body is always making the decision of what level of attention to engage when we go inside, we don't really know what will come forth.

Most people have a lot of opinions about "good" emotions they like to feel and "bad" emotions they don't think they're supposed to feel. So, sometimes, energy patterns can get trapped, clear down at the cell level. Let's say you're breathing, and an old memory comes up. You see yourself as a child pouting in the corner, feeling sad and neglected. Some part of you is still there, feeling sad and neglected and the last thing you want to do is to stir up all the pain that's been numbed away for years.

However, right now, in this meditative moment, you can go on a rescue mission and bring that child to safety. Go in and shout, "Run for your life!" and grab his or her hand and get 'em to safety. In this very moment, you're safe, right? So, in this moment by staying absolutely present with the breath you can go into a previous moment from this new place and it may shift.

Experience the shift as a felt experience. Breathe with what's going on now. If your body feels relief from this, be sure you sit with that and have the experience of relief. You want to integrate and stabilize the new pattern.

You can also go into the feelings evoked in difficult memories with compassion. You sit with the experience of sadness. You make room for it as holding a part of your precious humanity. You listen for its message as an expression of need, of what you care about, of what really matters to you. A soul song comes from this and you sing for other people who are glad for your company. If you allow a larger spaciousness around the experience and bring the breath toward it, you can begin a transformative process by which there is resolution at a new level.

The coyote howls at the moon, longing for something, and we too, howl for something we hope for, for something we lost, for something in ourselves to come to peace. Howling and howling. Then just because we showed up to do this, without warning, there is some new awareness, some new freedom, the minor key turns to the major resolution, or some release happens that allows for the energy held in a constricting pattern to become available for other uses. You may find that while the memory of the trauma is still there, it no longer holds you in the same way. And…this is also happening in the cell: energy has been released and made available for living with greater ease, freedom, and creativity, while holding greater compassion for yourself and others.

Traveling in this realm for healing purposes, especially where trauma is stored, can open new pathways and soothe old ones that are suffering from "hurt feelings." You have the gift of the breath to offer the cells over and over. The breath knows how to heal things. You don't have to know it all. Just take the breath into the body, into the sensations you experience, into the cells.

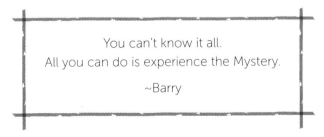

You can't know it all.
All you can do is experience the Mystery.

~Barry

Among the more poignant emotions is grief. Ahh! When grief arises, it too has a place in the body. Meeting this place, which the body reveals, with the mercy of the breath helps grief find the very alchemy by which healing actually happens even more deeply. This is different than thinking, "I just have to be cheerful."

On the contrary, you may find some very deep transformation by staying carefully present while the body is howling in lament, breathing into that, into the sensations, going into them just as you can with the breath, the merciful and powerful breath. You are staying present with the actual sensations in the body as the cells are transforming into greater intelligence. Often, as something new is trying to emerge, something old has to die. Saying goodbye may bring up grief. If this is what is alive in the cell community, we listen for the sensations in the body that want and need the Merciful Breath.

Once, I was in a very contracted state of grief after the death of my husband. Barry heard this and said, "Put on your raincoat and go outside where there is something larger than your grief." This was not the soothing comfort I was hoping for, since I was feeling sorry for myself and wanted sympathy, but I did put on my raincoat and I did go out in the gentle rain. I walked with the tears of the sky, and my grief did shift into greater peace. I had forgotten about the Great Space and letting it in, but Barry reminded me. Over the days and months that followed, I had his guidance pointing me toward looking for and opening myself to something greater, something "larger than my grief" to help me through the alchemical transformation that comes from being present to grief. Yes, our lives are often radically transformed by this profound emotion. Breath by breath, we receive exquisite care as we are being taken apart and reordered for whatever is to follow in our lives.

Breathing with joy
(and my feet begin to dance)
Howling with lament
(and my heart breaks open)
Roaring with anger
(and my confusion is burned to ashes)
Crouching in shame
(and my groveling shape-shifts to dignity)
Ha!
You just never know what the
Great Mystery
will send
for your soul's release.

Stay present with the feeling no matter what it may be.

I remember meditating with a woman who was overweight.

The sweetness of "orange" came to me in that moment.

I had compassion with the feeling.

I knew it was true because it resonated.

~Barry

9

Being IN the Body—
The Five Senses and Beyond

"A man will be imprisoned in a room with a door that's unlocked and opens inward, as long as it does not occur to him to pull rather than push."

~Ludwig Wittgenstein, philosopher
(1889–1951)

By now, it should be obvious that Cell Level Meditation is directed toward being in the body. You are actually tuning into the body as an expression of creativity, vitality, health, and human experience. Many people think they're supposed to have far-out experiences or see celestial beings. And nothing like this happens. Well, of course, it can and does happen, but that's not what we're aiming toward.

Can you be present for exactly what is going on, just as you experience it? Can you stay with the breath as it travels inside your nose? Can you experience the pause between the in-breath and the out-breath? Can you stay "conscious" as you experience the sensation in your nose as the breath goes all the way out? If you can do this, you are a Zen Master!

And, it's also true, that as you turn your awareness into your body, you can, over time, have an experience—either visual, auditory, or felt—of different body tissues. How the cells, organs and tissues make themselves known to you is just your unique way of perceiving things. Notice what comes to you, as it comes to you, stay with the sensations as they show up and breathe with them.

Since you have identified a certain intention or purpose for doing the meditation, let your breath go toward the place in your body that needs some breath. If you are working on the bones, take the breath into the bones. If you are working on the skin, take the breath into the skin. If you are working on healthy kidneys, take your breath into the kidneys. And so on.

So many things can happen as you do Cell Level Meditation. Sometimes, people think they can't meditate. Or they have ideas that they're supposed to see things or have certain experiences.

You just never know what's going to happen.

The first time I went into my liver cells, everything turned bright orangey-yellow. Now this is a color that is associated with bile, something the liver makes. In herbal medicine, some of the plants that are known to help the liver are bright yellow, like the dandelion! So, I had a good time, being fully alive to the experience of "yellow!" Yellow and what it evoked, and I breathed together.

A few people I've known have also had the experience of finding themselves "seeing" or "feeling" a certain color. By taking the breath into the color, we help the cells that seem to need that particular experience. The color energizes them or soothes them or tones them or helps them get rid of junk they don't need. So, if a color comes to you, stay present to your own experience of seeing it, sensing it, feeling the color's effect on you, and breathing into it. Dive into it. Have a full experience of it.

Now each color has its particular gifts and qualities. It is a manifestation of a frequency of the light spectrum. You can find out about these frequencies yourself, by letting yourself open to the experience of them in your own way.

Blue

I write.

I look for the bluest blue
a winged blue
the most maritime
the blue alone
most encrusted in its blueness.

I look for the bluest blue
the most exquisite blue for my tongue
the blue that joins all the blues written in space
the blue that was here
when the wolf opened his eyes.

I look for the bluest blue
the most inexorable
the widest of all schools of fish blue
I look for the bluest trill, that converts all bluish trills
into one single blue note.

I look for the bluest blue
that will make me shudder
in one eternal phrase, of blue.

I write...

~Ekiwah Adler-Beléndez, poet

Another thing cells like to experience is sound. As you are traveling inside yourself on the wings of your breath, you may hear a kind of sound. Maybe it's a high-pitched buzz or a low-pitched hum. Listen carefully. Let yourself fully experience that tone. Match your own voice to it if you can. Breathe into that sound and *with* the sound. Maybe you'll find yourself singing "The Blues!" Maybe that is the only sound that expresses your experience, and by fully being present for it, your body gets the one message it needs to order itself.

One time, a very interesting meditation came out of a song that mysteriously came to me. So, I breathed the song: "By the waters of Babylon, I sat down and wept, and wept…" Guess which cells were wanting attention that day? Yes! The bladder cells got my attention by singing a "water song."

Hey! Muscle Cell!

What do you want?

"Humm, humm, humm!"

So, I breathe,

"Humm, humm, humm!"

We are all breathing,

"Humm, humm, humm."

As I do this, I notice a kind of enlivening. The color I'm seeing (in my mind's eye) becomes brighter. There is a kind of joyfulness. "Humm. Humm. Humm." You just never know what the cells are going to want on any given day!

Later that day, you may be surprised to hear a song on the radio that makes you feel enlivened. Go ahead! Experience the enlivening as a sensation in the body. Now you can actually dance if you wish or move with the rhythm of the song if you wish, but if that's not possible, you can experience the "micro-movements" in your body as your cells are dancing. You may think this is all in your mind. Good! The mind and the body are dancing! Breathe with the music, the rhythm, the sensations of "micro-dancing" in the body. "Humm. Humm. Humm."

Actually, one of the best things you can do for yourself is to find your rhythm! One trauma specialist, Bessel van der Kolk M.D., thinks the main problem with trauma is that people lose their rhythm because during trauma our bodies can go into "fight, fright or freeze." This can be so overwhelming that the cells are moving too fast, too slow, or not at all! And they get stuck there, in a pattern that is not natural or healthy to them! So, listen attentively for the tones and music of your inner intelligence, and by all means, get your rhythm back.

Once I found myself "frozen" in disbelief at something shocking that had happened to me. Twenty years later, during meditation one day, I found myself "as if I were a stone." So, I experienced "stony-ness." I was shocked to discover that by allowing myself to experience this fully, the experience of pain and resentment seemed to dissipate … after 20 years, after lots of therapy, after every good intention in the book to forgive the person. Experiencing myself as "stone," was something that never occurred to me to do, and by simply being present for this, this too, it was the key in the lock to release me from a difficult situation.

As my body "unfroze," my own natural rhythm began to return. This was so counter-intuitive to me, but sometimes, to get where we'd like to be, we go by the way where we don't like to be.

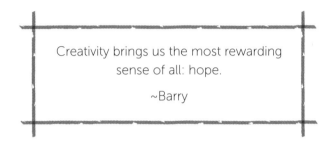

Creativity brings us the most rewarding sense of all: hope.

~Barry

Taste is another sense that the cells may use to get your attention. I have noticed that people have certain cravings for things that the cells need. So, if you discover the sensation of chocolate being alive in the body, that's the door in. Let the experience of the flavor be present. Enjoy it. Breathe it and then … become the sensations you're given. Once I was in the hospital and could not eat for about ten days. I spent a little time each day, fantasizing about lobster. Then I got really good at bringing forth from memory the experience of eating lobster, the texture, the flavor, the smell, the delight of this delicious food. A month later, when I was well and out of the hospital, my friends had a lobster dinner for me. It was great (but I confess, it wasn't as wonderful as the lobster I had in my meditations in the hospital)! Who knew that lobster would bring healing my way?

The sense of smell is said to evoke our deepest memories. Now it's true that the places our bodies want healing are stored in different levels of consciousness, or frequencies. Allowing ourselves to go deeply into the places in our cells where healing happens requires a letting go into altered states, almost like we're dreaming but participating in the dream. So, if you find a smell arising, sniff your way into that place and allow it to show you where it wants a breath of fresh air! Go into the aroma, breathe in the beautiful roses that are bringing a Valentine present to your heart, and become that, let the reality of it come forth in you as you breathe.

As you are breathing into your body, as you're paying attention to what's going on in your body, your five senses are speaking to you. Images or colors (visual) may appear in your mind's eye; buzzing sounds may become prominent or the memory of a beautiful piece of music or your cat may meow (use everything!); or a smell seems to waft by or evokes a memory of a scenario you need to revisit; or you become aware of a certain flavor; you notice a tingle, a twitch or a rhythmic throb, a slight pressure, the feel of velvet or prickly heat.

Notice, my friends, these are sensations in the body! We all have them! Just tune into what's there. Take your curiosity and awareness to what you actually experience. Allow yourself to be exquisitely present for this experience. (Try not to analyze it or draw premature conclusions from it, which will take you into the disconnected-thought-thinking mind and out of the fullness of the actual experience.) Be present for the sensations as an experience. Become these sensations. Breathe. You may discover there's a lot more there than you thought. How you experience it has to do with how you're put together. Breathe to that, to the Whole of you, containing and ordering all these flavors, colors and melodies, bringing them together in coherence, unfolding as a symphony that plays your very own song.

We have considered that we have five senses that help us experience the world. In meditation, something happens, in which we shift into a different "state" of awareness, where the five senses seem to have some numinous quality that deepens our experience of wonder. We get the sense, like a sixth sense, that there's something beyond what meets the eye (or the ear, nose, taste, touch or feel of things). By noticing the sensations in the body with curiosity, being present with them and breathing with them again and again, it may feel like you're going into a dream-world. In fact, the electrical frequencies in which your brain works when you are awake may change, like they do when you're dreaming. (Researchers have hooked electrodes to the scalps of really good meditators, and sure enough, their brainwaves change when they meditate! This can be measured!)

And of course, the nerves travel all over the body from … the brain, so the body, receiving signals from the meditating brain, can respond, and change, and heal—this is a good story for your thought-thinking mind. Cell Level Meditation may be compared with Lucid Dreaming, in which you, the Dreamer, are actually participating in the Dream. "You" are staying awake for the dream of the body, learning to perceive within a new frequency or "bandwidth of information storage." Your body stores things in all kinds of ways.

Like a ripple
That chases the slightest caress
Of the breeze—
Is that how you want me
To follow you?

~Ono No Komachi, Japanese Poet
(ca. 834–?)

Have you ever awakened with a vivid dream just as the phone was ringing? You spring out of bed and answer the phone. Your awareness shifts into your waking state, and you carry on a conversation with the caller. After the phone call, you can't remember the dream. Poof! It's gone! It was so vivid, and now it's gone. If you wanted to find the dream again, you would have to shift back into the frequency or state of awareness, like the channel you were in when you were in the dream. It turns out we're multi-dimensional beings with many levels of information stored in different levels and layers of awareness.

Many philosophers and neuroscientists have pointed out that there are three great states of awareness: Waking, Dreaming and Dreamless sleep. Each of these great states is correlated with a certain kind of awareness. As I mentioned, the neuroscientists can measure what's happening in the brain when we are in any of these states, by looking at the electric patterns of brain activity. And it's been said, that in the Waking State, only about 5% of our adult awareness is participating. The other 95% is "unconscious" to us, except by entering into altered states of awareness, in which we find a doorway into other levels of information storage.

By learning to enter into meditative states, we are shifting awareness to find the right door, the right frequency, the state where information is stored. Some people have found great value in working with a hypnotherapist who is trained to take people into different states of awareness where hidden information, beliefs, life strategies and energy patterns are stored. No matter how much you use your thinking mind to tell your body to get better, if you don't have a connection with the deeper energetic patterning, it may not be too effective.

Keep this in mind as you keep awareness "light" enough to find the frequency or state of mind your healing intention requires. With a connection to Silence (allowing for deep stillness), to the Breath, to your Heart's Desire, the body shifts its state, and little by little your thought-thinking mind moves out of the way and you enter into the state you need.

As we adopt a meditation practice, an embodied meditation practice, we actually change our level of being or how we participate in life, over time. Little by little we practice moving beyond our habitual "thought-thinking mind" to our "caring mind" to our "body-mind" to our "curious mind," and we are transformed. Our "senses" are objects of attention given to us as gifts to enliven our lives creatively.

And I will mention, it's not as difficult as you may think to tune into these mysterious places. When children were asked what love is, Bobby, age 7, said:

> "Love is what's in the room with you at Christmas
> if you stop opening presents and listen."

Yeah! Like that!

We get quiet and listen…the love is already there.

10

Standing Back Far Enough or High Enough to See

"Every man takes the limits of his own field of vision for the limits of the world."

~Arthur Schopenhauer, philosopher
(1788–1860)

Now, it's true, most of us have a bit of a challenge when we first sit down and try to become still to meditate. In our culture, we engage our thought-thinking minds so much, it can be hard to turn them off. Some Buddhists refer to this "chatty" quality of our thought-thinking minds as "The Monkey Mind." So, another useful skill is developing the ability to watch "the show" or to become witness to the thoughts.

It's true that the Monkey Mind can take over, and you just get too fidgety to meditate once in a while, so, you may have to get up and go do something else and come back to it later. But! I have another clue for you! Take a step back from "Monkey Mind." Notice that something in you (our friend, Awareness) can watch your mind jumping around, thinking of this and that. You stand back from the picture to "see" it from a larger perspective. From this perspective, notice the "quality" of what's going on. Notice the "jumping-around-from-subject-to-subject-quality." Or notice the random "going-all-over-like-a-pinball-machine-quality." Notice the overall sensation of this as you begin to see what's going on in your body. Can you sit with that sensation? Can you find where the sensation is most prominent in your body? If so, take the breath to it. See if it will let you in and join it with the breath.

- Breathe into "scattered."

- Breathe into "floating all over."

- Breathe into "can't settle down."

People are often surprised how familiar this sensation is. One man told me that his thoughts seemed random and that he couldn't concentrate. I told him to breathe into that. He was so surprised that this very sensation was so familiar to him—he never thought of going into it, since he'd spent so much of his life trying to avoid it. As he began to breathe toward what he described as "randomness," he found the door into a deeper level of experience. And, perhaps it won't surprise you to learn that he discovered this kind of "randomness" further on down the line in his meditations…and his cells.

It is different to get lost in something like "randomness" than to go into it intentionally. Sometimes you have to bring yourself back gently to your intention or go back to the breath to stay in a meditative state and not just fall asleep. It is pretty common to get lost now and then. Remember: notice the sensations, experience the sensations as they come to you, take the breath into the sensations, become the sensations, and keep breathing. With each breath you and your cells are discovering each other, negotiating, learning, communicating, and getting to know each other. Something greater is trying to emerge, and this is how it happens for you.

Watching the "show" of your thoughts, which come and go, helps you to develop an aspect of awareness that is sometimes called the Witness. This is a feature of Awareness that allows you to stand back and just observe. This can give you the larger perspective I just described, so you can take the breath to a larger movement that goes on inside of you. If you can develop this capacity and teach The Witness to be respectful of the body, you are really moving along. Even The Witness, thinking it's being objective, can take on habits very quickly. So, even the Great Witness … yet another level of Discerning Awareness … can teach the Witness to be kind and curious!

I am going to describe a scenario that you have probably encountered if you've ever tried to do any meditation at all. You sit down to meditate and right away your disconnected-thought-thinking mind kicks in with all kinds of thoughts, commentary and lists of things to do. Now the "Witness" is asked to notice not just the thoughts, but also the quality behind the thoughts and the sensations in the body where this quality might be identified. The minute you sit down to meditate, the disconnected-thought-thinking mind often shows up. You are breathing, in and out, and suddenly up on the screen of the mind comes a thought:

"Oh, I must remember to get bread at the store."

Now there probably isn't a lot of emotional charge associated with this thought, so you can just notice it showed up and go back to breathing, in and out, in and out. Then another thought comes:

"Oh, also soap, I need to get soap."

And on the heels of this thought, another thought intervenes, saying:

> "You idiot! Can't you just shut up and be silent? You're supposed to be meditating, damn it!"

Now, if we step back in these easy-to-imagine scenarios, there is a feeling or a felt sense about each one, no? In the first thought, there's probably not a lot of energy or "charge." You probably don't have strong feelings about such a thought, right? So, in the body, things are still fairly neutral. Not much is going on. In the second thought, the judgmental thought, there might be quite a bit of energy. It may evoke strong feelings. These feelings show up as an experience in the body. Where is this energy in the body? Is there tightness in the jaw? Tension in the shoulders? Wherever and whatever the sensation is, experience that. Become that sensation. Take the breath to it.

This is the active part of the meditation. You're not falling asleep; you're not being swept away in your usual thought processes; you're noticing and sensing exactly what comes to you, the feeling in the body or how you perceive it. Then, you go into it. You take the breath into it. You become it. You are going beyond the thoughts, into the underlying experience of energy in the thoughts as it lives in your body, diving in through the place beyond your mind.

And, guess what? All of this happens at the cell level. You experience the cells in the best way your psyche knows how to get your attention!

The Guest House

This being human is a guest house
Every morning a new arrival.

A joy, a depression, a meanness,
Some momentary awareness comes
As an unexpected visitor.

Welcome and entertain them all!
Even if they're a crowd of sorrows,
Who violently sweep your house
Empty of its furniture,

Still, treat each guest honorably.
He may be clearing you
Out for some new delight.

The dark thought, the shame, the malice,
Meet them at the door laughing,
And invite them in.

Be grateful for whoever comes,
Because each has been sent
As a guide from beyond.

–Rumi, Persian poet and mystic
(1207–1273)

Our development is such that each step leaves an imprint. We slog through...We leave traces of our developmental process through energy. When these traces become fixated, they form constellations.

There are energy sources, different ones at different times that go back and perceive what was happening, even in utero. We uncover memories and find an energy constellation chart from atomic explosions that are traumatic, like in situations of rape or incest, PTSD.

We have a story that goes with this. We can see the defense mechanism that became a strategy to survive. Each of us can see these patterns; they are like stars in the body. If events are recalled, we see where the energy is lit up.
We can then shift this energy.

If we want to deal with the energy, not the story about an event, we have to deal with what is intangible in terms of physics.

~Barry

11

Meditating with Nature

Watching the moon
At dawn,
Solitary, mid-sky,
I knew myself completely,
No part left out.

~Izumi Shikibu, Japanese poet
(970–?)

Turning the attention to something larger than yourself, something you recognize as already Whole and beautiful and good, helps you remember and realign with your own Wholeness (the word from which "health" comes). Great herbalists report being able to tune into a plant and to ask it what it heals. Being a little denser than these great healers, I have to fall back on my experience of nature. Looking at a plant, I get silent. Then I notice what response I get in my body by gazing on this plant. What sensations can I notice? Sometimes, I have to become more silent (go deeper into no-thing) before I can notice what sensations the plant evokes in me. I breathe into this sensation.

One spring, I discovered a deep sense of calm by breathing toward the velvety darkness in the inner chamber of a tulip. Over the next few days, I found myself going back to this velvety silence that I experienced as calming and soothing, and my whole body would become relaxed and peaceful. What a gift that tulip gave me!

Then, one autumn, I got a very bad cough, and my trachea, or windpipe, felt very irritated. I realized after a week or so that I was very drawn to admire the pine trees as they lined up along the roads where I live. I breathed with the trees and noticed my windpipe seemed to enjoy it. But there's more—without really thinking about it, I was determined to line my driveway with two-foot logs, standing up, to make a little barrier between the gravel and the grass.

It didn't occur to me what my psyche was up to until I happened to be reading about columnar cells in an anatomy textbook. It turns out that there are cells in the trachea that are standing up in columns (columnar cells) and they kind of guard this tube into the lungs by helping stop dust particles and bacteria. Aha! Maybe that's why I'd been breathing toward the trees and making little stand-up barriers. Certainly, the irritation eased off and I got better. Maybe my columnar cells were inspired to stand up straighter!

In nature (and in our lives) there is usually something right in front of us, reminding us, showing us how healing is coming about in our bodies. So, look around and see what you are drawn to breathe into.

Your mind-body loves metaphors
It's a poet, you know.
It likes seeing how one thing is like another,
Like how tall pines along the road
Are like the columnar cells
Along the road to the lungs.
Breathe to that!

You may be a sensitive person. Perhaps you have developed an above-average level of perception and have the experience that we actually inhabit a Living and Responsive World, an Ensouled Cosmos! Maybe you are like Saint Francis of Assisi, who was a nature mystic. He was able to participate in the created universe as a living being with Brother Sun, Sister Moon, Brother Air, and Sister Water. He gave us a way to be in deeper connection with them:

Our Hands imbibe like roots
so I place them on what is beautiful in this world.

And I fold them in prayer, and they
draw from the heavens
light.

~St. Francis of Assisi, mystic
(1182–1226)

Let's make room for you to enjoy your sensibilities and align with them for your own healing. Go into Nature and notice your response, what you actually experience. Most of us have to get out of our heads to open up to this experience these days because many people are "nature deprived." That's ok. You know what I'm going to say, right? Notice the sensations in your part of nature, your body. Notice you are having an experience. Maybe it is subtle. Maybe you can enhance it by mimicking the shape of a plant or the posture of an animal. Let your own body experience this. Just stay with it, play with it, breathe with it in curiosity. In my part of the country, there is a lot of criticism about "Tree Huggers." Don't worry, you can go and hug a tree and see what your experience is, and I won't tell anyone. I'll let you tell them what you discovered. The natural world is alive, and enlivening. It has already solved the problem of keeping dust out of the lungs by creating "columnar cells," so if you listen and find a way to perceive what's there, you may receive very healing gifts.

"[In nature there is] beauty you feel in your flesh. You feel it physically, and that is why it is sometimes terrifying to approach. Other beauty takes only the heart, or the mind."

~Barry Lopez, environmentalist

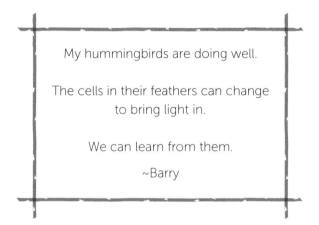

My hummingbirds are doing well.

The cells in their feathers can change
to bring light in.

We can learn from them.

~Barry

12

Resistance

"A clash of doctrines is not a disaster—it is an opportunity."

~Alfred North Whitehead, philosopher
(1861–1947)

Sometimes you may find yourself irritable, skeptical, and doubtful. Oh, these clever tricksters who try to keep you from your heart's desire! Now you may have to be even more clever than they are, on occasion! You may have to put on your coyote skin and, unnoticed, slink by the monster that says, "You can't do this!" You may have to tiptoe by him or slip by when his back is turned. You may have to say, "No!" and experience the strength of your clarity and dignity.

Some people are able to take the breath to these feelings, however. I knew one young man who was very aware of not wanting to get well. He felt embarrassed to admit it, but every time he had to do physical therapy, he just came up against his resistance. So, one day, he decided to explore it. He found the resistance in his body and took the breath right to it. He breathed into the resistance. Before long, he found himself in a meditative state, floating around in water, and it was quite blissful. Suddenly, boom! The water rushed out and he was being born…prematurely. He was so angry with that! He really wanted to be back in that blissful, warm water of his mother's womb. You know what he did? He spent several sessions in the bliss of the water. He found it calmed something in him and the resistance to doing the physical therapy decreased.

As you may notice from reading about this fellow's resistance or remembering some experience you've had with –

Not Wanting Things To Be The Way They Are

you may notice there can be a lot of energy stored in this. Since part of our job is to notice where the energy is stored and to decide if it's serving our well-being or not, first you must notice that this is so. Just noticing that you're really having an inner tantrum about –

Not Wanting Things To Be The Way They Are

may be liberating. This tantrum may be stored more as a "whine." Why me? Just feel the "why me?" That's resistance.

I remember another young man with a lot of psychological training. He had a good measure of insight into himself, and these insights sometimes turned into excuses that didn't really serve him all that well. He discovered an idea he had that he was "too hard on himself." Trying to counter this "idea," gave him an excuse to stay in bed every morning in a way that left him a little lethargic all day. His resistance to getting up at a time which allowed him to take a walk wasn't really serving him, since he'd discovered through his own experiments that he felt better and had more energy when he actually got up and got his walk in. So, "too hard on himself" was an idea, a disembodied thought. It wasn't really connected to Truth.

The actual experience, in the body may be another way through to a deeper aliveness. In his case, he discovered at times, he needed to be a little harder on himself!

I know another woman who was able to be very honest about her resistance to getting well. She discovered there was actually a benefit to being sick since it put her in contact with care and caring people! She felt a lot of shame about this discovery. People can say cruel things, like "You're just doing this to get attention." And then, we demonize a genuine need for attention (or an old need of our inner three-year-old). So, there was unresolved tension in her between wanting health and wanting care. These are both lovely concerns, no? So, this "resistance to getting well," brought up the tension, and the tension was the meditation.

Another example of using resistance to help you, is to acknowledge the experience of it instead of judging yourself or suppressing it — we want the energy from everything! I went to visit a friend's mother, who was in the hospital after a stroke. This lovely Jewish woman, who was 92, had always been quite spunky, but now she couldn't speak. When I sat down with her, she made a gesture of frustration. Had she been able to speak, I'm pretty sure she would have said, "Oy! Vey!"

Once she made this gesture that fully expressed not liking the way things were, she got quiet. A light came to her eyes. Somehow, using hand movements, she was able to let me know that I should get out paper and pencil. She couldn't write, but as I pointed to the letters of the alphabet I created on the page, she could nod when I had the letter she wanted, until she spelled out the words she wanted to communicate to me! Amazing!

I have thought many times about this experience. The "discharge" or perhaps the full expression of her resistance, through that gesture, was like a clearing so she could solve the problem of communicating with me, using the tools still available to her!

Resistance, by nature and definition, slows things down. In our warp-speed society, this can be helpful to find a place in ourselves where we can acknowledge the many layers and levels of our lives. Sometimes our resistance shows us what needs to transform before we can move on. These things are pretty tricky. You can see how convoluted the path can be at times.

So, resistance? First find it. If you can acknowledge it, you can have an experience in "slowing down" and finding your truth.

And! Like Odysseus on his journey homeward, use every trick in the book!

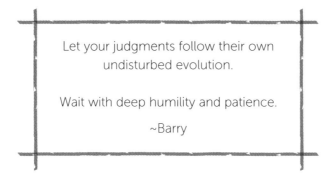

Let your judgments follow their own undisturbed evolution.

Wait with deep humility and patience.

~Barry

13

Breathing to Beliefs

"A belief is not merely an idea the mind possesses,
it is an idea that possesses the mind."

~Robert Bolton, author,
quoted in the London *Guardian* Newspaper

You may discover deep beliefs that seem to live (or possess you) in your body, all the way down to the level of the cells.

One woman I know, for example, inherited both the physical tendency and the mental tendency of perfectionism. In Cell Level Meditation, she got to the very core of this "structure" within herself. She found cells that were "perfect," absolutely sterile and mechanical. They were all the same.

She had before complained bitterly about her upbringing with a mother that treated her and her siblings in exactly the "same" way. They were all dressed alike, given the same foods to eat, and so on. Now, at the very core of her being she found the same tendency, expressed at a cellular level.

She had to breathe into her pain about that. She went into the cells and began to pay attention to them and to tune into what seemed good for them and to distinguish what felt right from what she habitually thought was right in a mechanical, perfectionist way. She was able to question her beliefs about conformity and perfectionism and become more fluid and creative in the moment's requirements of her.

Outwardly and inwardly there was more repertoire of response.

You may discover pain that needs to be healed, values you need to uphold, your strengths that make you bold, and your fears that take you down. And you discover what is truly healing as you take the breath to the cells. You may find something startlingly familiar as you find yourself traveling into the cells. You can ask yourself, "Where else have I experienced this?" Try not to get stuck in the story and keep breathing creatively. Distinguish between mind and body and bring breath to the body's sensations now. Experience those sensations. Try them on. Become those sensations. Breathe some more. Participate in the Mystery, instead of thinking about it. Dance, instead of thinking about which foot goes left, and which foot goes right.

You may find yourself angry about being sick or trying to find out why you're sick. Hey, you don't really know why you're sick. No one knows. Having an illness is so mysterious. But here it is. You want to get better. If you're angry about being sick, breathe into the anger! Mine the energy in the anger and use it to rally your healing response.

I worked with a fellow who had terrible problems with emphysema; he was shocked to discover something he couldn't let himself acknowledge. He really believed he was incurable. This was so hidden to him, since he'd spent years and lots of money on lots of different therapies, but there it was as plain as day when he breathed toward his lungs: a recalcitrant belief that he was incurable. I must say, in his case, he didn't have a lot of help from the collective belief system. Lots of people think emphysema is incurable. Now he didn't want to believe he was incurable, but this is what he found cemented into body and reinforced by everyone he knew. Frankly, we can't really sneeze at the Collective Belief System – it has a lot of power and has to be met with something of a "similar matching power" if it's taken hold in us.

Some of our most recalcitrant beliefs come to us when we are really young, before we have the kind of awareness you're using now in reading this. We are like sponges when we're little and take in "how the world works" from every cue that is given to us. In fact, something in us is receiving information while we're being born, already taking in the rules of the world – whether we're safe or not, whether the world is a good place or not. These beliefs are so deep you can't really get to them with your rational mind, but they seep into your life in all kinds of ways. I confess, this is actually one of the reasons I became a midwife! I wanted to save people from "bad information" that is imprinted on babies at birth.

Doing breathwork … especially with someone who can be present with you, can help you get into the "state of awareness" where this information is stored in you and became the basis of unquestioned beliefs about life you took on then.

If you find yourself believing your illness is some kind of punishment, notice where that lives in your body and breathe to that. Acknowledge your belief. Maybe you have to make amends somewhere. Or maybe you have to breathe to a belief that no longer serves you, and let it loosen its hold on you, and say, "Be gone!" Or (and most likely) just by experiencing the sensations fully, that is the key in the lock to release you! Whoa!

> "Dost thou think because thou art virtuous,
> there shall be no more cake and ale?"
>
> ~William Shakespeare

You may be surprised to find beliefs or emotions that are relics from the past, from your ancestors. One day, I discovered a deep sense of homesickness, and I had a brief glimpse of getting off a boat and feeling overwhelmed. My grandparents were immigrants to the US, and it came to me that this homesickness I've known all my life as a vague sense was something that possibly came down to me from my grandmother, whom I never met! (Oh, I see you are laughing that I started this book with a story about a guy who is trying to get home! There's just no hiding from ourselves, no?)

Everything that you can become aware of is a place for exploration, a place to discover, engage, experience, and toward which you can take the breath. Beware of getting caught up in analyses or explanations—just be honest with what you experience and ... breathe to the sensation it evokes in you in the body. Take healing breath, holy spirit, to the body and let it all come into healing. Get out of your own way!

In the process of doing this, you become a more vibrant expression of the life force that lives through you. Yes, you! You are the unique and creative expression of something very mysterious. Cell Level Meditation helps you discover yourself way down deep. Gradually, a sense of this marvelous life force that is you begins to evoke awe and respect. Then true self-confidence and self-esteem may be born. Not because you're supposed to have self-confidence, but because you have touched something inside yourself that you know is beautiful and wonderful, and quite naturally, you want to live in harmony with it. It feels real to you. You become a co-participant with Life, rather than a victim or a tyrant. This may happen because you are more conscious of what is true for you and have found a quality of awareness where you just know it. It is an experience and it is yours.

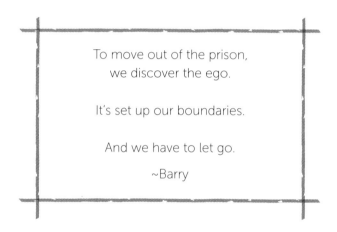

To move out of the prison,
we discover the ego.

It's set up our boundaries.

And we have to let go.
~Barry

14

Treatments and Medication, Vitamins and Herbs

"Because there is that sort of feeling that people don't know what to do with gaps in their lives. It's a scary notion, but actually, if you stand in space just for a little while, a new door will open, or you'll be able to see in the dark after a while. You'll adjust."

~Jane Campion, screenwriter
Quoted in www.quotemaster.org

Consider for a moment, that all kinds of messengers are arriving at the door of the cell, all the time. The cell can say, "Hey, come in," or, "Go away," or, "Come back later." While we often have the idea that this is a fairly mechanical process, there is something more at work…in the gap…where you can let the breath, a prayer, an intention, or words of encouragement in. So, if you are taking medications, a homeopathic remedy, vitamins, herbs or receiving some kind of treatment for an illness, use Cell Level Meditation to focus and enhance the treatment.

Take a few moments to get quiet and go into silence. Tune into your body. Tune into your intention for taking the medication or treatment. Let your body know that help for healing is on the way. Sense your body's response to this and breathe. Breathe to the cells, "Help is on the way!"

As you take the medication, use your breath to direct it to the purpose for which it's intended. Whisper in the ear of the attack dog, "Sic 'em! Go get those cancer cells (or viruses or bacteria or other bad-guys)!" Maybe you'll feel protective of your healthy cells. Listen in and breathe toward their protection. Shield them from any noxious side effects.

> Breath to cells.
> Breathe! Breathe! Breathe!
> You don't have to know how to do it all.
> Take in the breath, the Mighty Breath.
> May you benefit completely.
> May the benefit be great.
> May the benefit be completely great.
> May you have every assistance you need.

A teacher I knew made a trip around the world. He was a little nervous about getting sick in countries where sanitation systems weren't as sophisticated as he was used to. When he got to these countries, he would put his hands on his stomach before eating. He'd notify his body that food was coming and that lots of people ate this food and benefitted from it. He'd tune in and let his body know it could find a healthy relationship with the food. He never got sick.

This same man could also go to the vitamin section of a store and ask his body if any particular vitamin would benefit him. He could sense what he needed and what he didn't need. As you get better at tuning into yourself, this won't seem strange to you. Tune in and "listen" (sense, feel or "see," according to your way of tuning in) for your body's response to food, vitamins, medications and whatever else you take into yourself. Hmmm, sounds like a way to be more conscientious in general!

Working with a lovely woman who had cancer, after she
has shifted into a meditative state, I ask,
"What does the cancer cell look like?"

"It's like a square cinnamon roll, a kind of rounded square
with an orange nucleus."

"Can you go into it?"

"Yes, it's soggy in here, lifeless. It doesn't want to live.
It just wants to die."

"Is that a familiar feeling?"

"Oh yes! I have felt so drained of energy and lifeless. I can't
stand up and be myself. I have to keep myself small. I just
want to die sometimes. This is very familiar."

"Can you see any other healthy cells around it?"

She breathes and moves out of the cancer cell.

"Yes. I see them. They are vibrant and alive."

"What is their response to the cancer cell?"

She pauses, and then says,
"I see them coming around the cell with a kind of blanket;
there are four of them and they are bringing the 4 corners
of the blanket together to wrap it up to take it away."

"Can you become one of them?"

"Yes. I am alive, energized.
I feel sorry for the cancer cell, but I really don't need it
anymore.

I am done with it. R.I.P."

As we finish the session, she is worried she hasn't done it
right. But she says, she's never gotten this far, this deep,
nor felt this clear about the difference between her healthy
cells and the way she perceives the cancer cells. The
immune system doesn't always recognize unhealthy cells...
it's complex.

In this session, this woman was very clear by look, feel,
emotion and belief!

In the next session, we might begin to explore "doubt" and
how and where that lives in the system.

~Patricia

I know another woman who decided to get chemotherapy for cancer. She was very worried about the toxic effect of this treatment on the healthy cells of her body. She went into meditation, and gave her healthy cells little yellow rain slickers, so they would be protected from the "acid rain" of the chemotherapy. Whenever she went to get the infusion of chemotherapy, the healthy cells had their rain slickers on, and received protection. She had very few side-effects from chemotherapy, her choice of healing.

An interesting area in medical research is trying to determine the "placebo effect" from the "real effect" of a drug that is being studied for efficacy. The placebo effect is often spoken about in a derogatory way, associated with the idea "it's all in your head." Ah! But it is now known that what you think, what is in your "head," does affect things "downstream."

What you think and the way you think it does create the release of neurochemicals that give messages to your body about how it should respond to all kinds of things. We have already seen that there is a lively interaction between mind and body, between our perceptions of substances we take in and how our body receives them. There is, similarly, a "nocebo effect," which is what happens when you believe something you're taking is bad for you, and guess what? Your body has a negative response to it.

Barry spoke to me about a grant he'd received to help people who were receiving stem-cell transplants. If someone gets a transplant, their very clever body may reject the new cells as "foreign," and so they need drugs to keep their body from rejecting the new cells. Barry asked the nurses to meditate with the containers holding the stem cells before the transplant procedure. He asked them to love the little stem cells. Unfortunately, this little procedural detail was eliminated from the study because the researchers thought it was too weird. But Barry knew how to work with these cells. Awareness and intention for the good, for love, matters! They are part of a coherent field which influence an outcome.

However, I have another friend, who participated in a research study in which she meditated at a distance on a culture medium where bone cells were to be grown. She concentrated on this medium for five minutes, just loving it and sensing the holiness of life, and guess what? The bone cells grew better in that medium, a lot better, significantly better, than the ones grown in the "unloved" medium. Whoa! It seems quite practical to know that these minds of ours are potent! And what could we achieve with this knowledge!

When you are receiving care from people, hopefully, you will find people who are knowledgeable, skilled, helpful and holistic, to help you and guide you and encourage you and give you good medicine. Being open to receive help is useful. And being alert to your true sense of the relationship you have with each person is also wise. Get a second opinion if you experience dissonance or take the "good" and put your rain slicker on for where that "expert" can't quite validate what you know as a deep truth.

I knew of a woman who locked herself in a room to heal from a difficult disease. She had friends bring food to the door of her room, but she really wanted to learn to listen to the deep healing voice she had found within. She chanted, meditated, and tuned into this deep sense of herself she had discovered.

After a couple of months, she realized she was Whole. She sensed she no longer had the disease. However, when she imagined going to the doctor to corroborate her experience, she found fear and doubt. She knew she wouldn't be able to stay connected to this inner truth she had discovered if he countered her. So, she spent another month until she knew without a doubt that she had, in fact, healed. This was "gnosis," which is a kind of knowing that comes from true experience, not just ideas or wishful thinking. When this was truly her inner knowing, she did go to her medical doctor, and the tests did come back that showed she no longer had the disease.

Dr. Rocco Ruggiero, D.C., worked with Barry in Napa in the early days of developing this work. In a personal communication, he shared this insight:

"Most of the 'imagery practitioners' seemed to be intent upon intruding their notions of what the patient 'should' visualize in order to defeat one's disease. This was the mistake that Simonton made: taking the effective imagery that one patient created and offering that to another patient similarly afflicted. That might work with antibody production, but not with imagery work. So, rather than Guided Imagery we went to Unguided Imagery. I preferred the name Evoked Imagery work. 'E VOCA' means to elicit, to extract from the voice and the words of the patient.

As individuals were asked to describe their sense of the problem or condition, they usually would say something like, 'this is going to sound really crazy (weird, strange, bizarre) but it looks like, it seems like…' There was some sense that they couldn't say this any place else.

Then we would inquire if the image was ok with them. If not, what would they change? For that change to occur, did they have resources within themselves to resolve it? (If yes, we then would follow that out. If no, this might lead to the realization of a needs for another intervention such as chemotherapy. If chemo was required, we helped them find a better course through chemo.) Barry and I both saw cases where a well-intentioned therapist intruded into the patient's process rather than finding what was unique and true for that person.

This approach is ancient. Socrates did it in extracting the answers from the mouths of the questioners."

If you are going to receive something into your body, into your life, into your little cells, find the good in it. Bless it. Certainly, this causes no harm, and… it may do a lot of good.

15

Only One You—Creativity and Originality

"Flee with thy life if thou fearest oppression
and leave the house to tell its builder's fate.
Thou wilt find, for the land that thou quittest, another,
But no soul wilt thou find to replace thine own."

~One Thousand and One Nights,
Arabian folk tale

And you will also be creative! Be original. Go into everything with all of who you are. Try things on and throw them out. Notice what seems true to you! Just breathe to the cells, to the sensations you experience, to what you are aware of. Experience everything fully as your own experience. Just breathe! And, in your creativity, you may be moved to sing to your cells. I love lullabies, and as a mother or perhaps due to years of working with mothers and babies as a midwife, the feeling of tenderness lives in me. So, sometimes when I am breathing toward some cells that seem to want comfort, I sing a lullaby to them. I "breathe" the lullaby toward them. "There, there, little cells. Mom's here, you're going to be alright."

Do you like to dance? Once in a cell meditation I was exploring some feelings of anger I found in some cells, and on the magic carpet of the breath I brought in a troupe of Flamenco dancers to "match" the sense of outrage I discovered in my body. My cells really enjoyed that one! The cells have rhythm too!

A woman I worked with saw the black image of death that came to her in a meditation session. She couldn't get rid of it, so she told it to get to work on the cancer cells in her body. Pretty gutsy!

A young man, who was just discovering young women, had to work on the myelin sheaths around his nerves. He found himself imagining a beautiful girl pulling on her stocking.

If you are a miner, you might find yourself mining the energy from a pattern to make it available for something else. If you are an electrician, you might find yourself re-wiring the circuitry where the current is not running right.

Barry told me about a man he worked with who was an expert on the human eye. He was able to re-engineer his own eyes and regain his sight! Now that's focus! And he was quite motivated because he really wanted, just yearned to see the face of his wife.

Barry also had a client who breathed to his liver, and he discovered the liver was a factory. So, he found a way to make the factory work better.

Another woman Barry worked with had to create white blood cells to survive, and she set up a factory with the 7 dwarfs, who were singing all the time, "Whistle while you work."

As you explore all of these avenues of your own experience, my advice is to be creative, use your breath, and stay present with your own experience until you sense things are "in order" for that session. The great mystics tell us that "the most personal becomes the most universal."

Your part in the Grand Order of things is very personal and tied to Everything! Nevertheless, it is yours and yours alone.

How long does it take for things to heal? There is no simple way of answering this. A true healer would say things are already healed, and how long it takes you to remember that depends on your nature or fate or who knows? Things can heal in an instant! I know of one fellow who worked for three years to fully recover. Some cells in the body seem to act faster than others. Maybe it's easier to get into some kinds of body cells for you than for others. Some cells are speedy, and some are slow. Match the speed as you become the sensation. Maybe an instant healing would be too frightening for you because it would challenge everything that you hold dear, so it might be easier to heal a little at a time. Perhaps, our healing is impeded by our conditioning. If you've lived with something for a long time, you've made all kinds of allowances for this, and a pattern of compensation gets set up in the whole body, the nervous system, and the brain. You can have an amazing breakthrough, and then you may have to practice getting used to being healthy.

Once I healed a chronic knee problem and I noticed I was waiting for the problem to come back rather than enjoying and stabilizing the healed sensation. I had gotten so used to dealing with my bad knee that I didn't know how to be with my good knee. I had to practice. So, in the spirit of integration and the experience of being human, it seems like an on-going practice is useful for many people. It just seems to take time to get in, to integrate the experience, to make it solid and stabilize it, and to realize, "My God! This stuff works!"

"The fox has his den, and the bird has his nest,
but the Son of Man has nowhere to rest his head."

~Matthew 8:20

Being human, we are told there is no dogma that can tell us how to meet every situation that comes up. But we do have the breath! That's the great tool in this meditative practice. And that brings us back to the Mystery, back to the spaciousness around us. Our own lives have come out of that Mystery, and can be healed, reprogrammed, and realigned when we turn toward a sense of newness to every moment by watching, listening, sensing into the situation, and diving in with our own instincts and awareness and delight. Of course, you will discover this on your own. Perhaps you will try using something that "worked" for you yesterday, and today it flops. Or maybe it won't!

There's just no dogma that always works, no place to rest your head. You are unique and different among all people. Whatever you are given is yours to bring to the moment. This is a paradox. On one hand, I'm suggesting that you come to the meditation, breath or moment with newness and freshness, and on the other, I'm telling you to bring all of who you are to the moment. Yes, both of these statements are useful tools! There is just no place where we can rest our heads!

In general, I would venture to say, that we must get out of our "heads" when we do Cell Level Meditation.

In fact, it's the most important thing you can do!

Instead of analyzing your experience, be present for the experience, go into it as an experience. Breathe into it. Simply wonder. Many things will come to you to engage: dreams, thoughts, beliefs, emotions, memories, visual images, sounds, smells, and so on. Instead of thinking about what comes to you or wondering "why or how or what does it mean," my best advice is to ask, "Where is it in the body?" Go into the sense of it (as it comes to you), experience what comes to you, take the breath into it and enter into as an actor in your own play, become that, and let it come to fullness. We're all curious about why things are the way they are. (And, as I mentioned, the "whys" can get you!) If we go into our heads too fast, we may not find out the deeper, more satisfying answers that end up connecting us way beyond what we could imagine. So, if you find yourself in very familiar territory, notice that it's familiar, and keep going!

Somehow, it's what you care about the most deeply, that is your greatest gift. Opening your true heart into that leads you to what's alive in you. It's a felt sense, an intuition that's in the body. It's stored in you, in that place where you feel wonder. It's hard to put words on it. Poets allude to it. Artists show us the light of it. Maybe, if you're a mathematician, you can express it in an equation! When an equation is true, the mathematician is thrilled: Eureka! Barry called it Beauty.

Because our bodies and all their cells are tuned to different ways of knowing, many people can find what they care about by breathing and feeling the breath in the chest. The physical heart is in the chest, and opening into the way the spiritual heart "speaks" takes you to an experience of care, kindness, dare I say, "love?" If you can drop from head (thoughts) to heart (what you love), you will notice that your awareness shifts. Can you experience the delight, the sheer delight of being in the field of love? You can't really negotiate love, but you can experience it as a guiding light to what truly matters to you. Breathe with that.

First, acknowledge the Mystery.
There is an ultimate Seer.
There is only One.

Some people are able to access a path or sense
a vibration.
I call it Beauty.

Some can access Beauty more in its totality.
These people are guides / mentors.
Hopefully, they are honest.

Many people are able to access "partial beauty."
Some people access only a little.
Some people, none.

We've been told we have to access all or none.
This isn't true.

When there is fear, we access less beauty.
Some people challenge us to access more beauty,
like Mozart.
But, if we come away with less, it's OK.

The greatest struggle of humankind is thinking
we have to be more.

We don't trust our sense of things.
Just turn your sense into accepting beauty,
as it comes to you.

~Barry

16

Experiencing the Cells

"Go sit in your cell and your cell will teach you everything."

~Ascribed to one of the Desert Fathers,
Christian monks in the Scetes Desert of Egypt

And you may be wondering, but what about the cells? This is Cell Level Meditation! Yes, we can get all the way down to the cells. In fact, anything that you are doing or thinking is also, in some way, going on in the cells, no? It's already happening, and you are learning to shift into states of awareness in which you can be co-creative and engaged with what's already going on!

A woman I know got to the bone cells, and what most surprised her is that they were doing their "bone cell thing" independently of what she thought or said or did. We might say, the bone cells already know what to do! Thankfully so!

Everything ultimately is a pattern of energy in expression. The manifest form, if you travel into it, is made of smaller parts, the smaller parts are made of even smaller parts, and so on, until you get down to a level where there is only the sensation of something like vibrancy itself arising from the emptiness.

The expression of the energy of a substance running at a certain rate is solid, at another rate it's liquid, and at another it's a gas. Every known substance has its parameters, temperature, rate and rhythm, and how it behaves under different circumstances.Similarly, different types of cells in the body have their own "signature" pattern of color, movement, speed, sound, or energetic frequency. Muscle cells have a different kind of pattern than bone cells. And they "feel" different than bone cells in some kind of subjective way. The cells are working along with their own programming, and if you are suffering from an illness, you might find a sense of unease or disturbance when you get there. How do we work with that? Breathe to it! Experience it as it comes to you and be with it!

Become it! Be responsive. Just keep breathing. Stay curious and simply wonder how to engage the experience fully, looking for clues. It seems counter-intuitive to "become the disease," but you may have a sense that you will find the road to healing mysteriously revealed to you by doing just that.

Now because I have worked in health care, I have had to study such things as biology and anatomy and physiology. So, I have seen the pictures of cells in textbooks and under the microscope. However, the first time I "saw" the cell membrane in Cell Meditation, I was quite moved. It was much more dynamic than I had imagined, and beautiful! A few years later, I was delighted to see a photo of a cell membrane taken with the use of an electron microscope. I was excited to have my vision corroborated. A couple of times I have had something like this happen, a beautiful confirmation.

Once I got to a structure in my body that somehow, I identified as a virus. It was very resistant to being in relationship with the other cells. In fact, it felt very "other," or foreign to me. And, it was quite a rascal! A few weeks later, I went to pick up a friend at a doctor's appointment. While I was in the waiting room, waiting for her, I picked up a magazine, and there on the cover was a picture of the virus I'd seen, taken under an electron microscope!

Sometimes (actually, most of the time), I've noticed that the "cellular picture" comes as a metaphor. For example, one patient I work with has some problems with her cholesterol levels, and when she went in, she described to me some pipes. As her description became more vivid and dynamic, I realized she was in the cardiovascular system, working on the plaque on the wall of blood vessels that needed some attention.

Other times, some people I've worked with have gone into the structure of the cell. There is a kind of geometry with shapes, color, movement, and vibrancy. Participating in the harmony and beauty of this underlying pattern is an experience of great delight.

I know people who have a disciplined Qigong practice. Qigong is a centuries-old system of coordinated body posture and movement, breathing, and meditation used for the purposes of health, spirituality, and martial arts training. Through a focused use of their whole bodies people who practice this discipline learn a sense of rhythm and flow of movement that brings harmony to the body and peace to the mind. These very people bring their Qigong practice into the cells, where they sense a micro-movement at a more subtle level of inner experience. When a cell within a tissue, within an organ is not functioning well, there is a subjective experience that something is "off." The people who have this practice become very good at moving their awareness within and entering into the on-going dialogue with their embodied selves. They practice inner Qigong "re-minding" the cells of their innate rhythm and harmony.

And! The potential that lies within you may astound you! The cells of the body are quite versatile, noble, and capable of transformation (just like you are)! We have already mentioned stem cells. These are cells that haven't been programmed yet for a specific job.

We become aware that the cells turn over and that some cells can become any other cell.

A cell can go into neutral entropy. It can transform.

It becomes the new cell.

Breathe with it and allow it to have the experience of itself as a new cell with itself.

Then let it have the experience of the Whole.

~Barry

Cells might be considered as an archetypal template for life. They are the smallest unit of life. Life, by its very nature is … alive! Because it is alive, it is not just responding in a set, mechanical way, but rather it is responsive to what is needed and helpful and useful. Once they are given a job, a function, they take on an identity and leap into the cell community as participants in life.

Whatever you can imagine, opens possibilities that can birth into physical reality. The noble cells of your body can rest, take stock of the situation, and create solutions to problems. They can transform. They use creative solutions. In addition to their versatility, what makes the cells of the body so successful is their ability to cooperate! Sounds like we should be taking classes from them.

Barry offers us a wonderful breathing meditation for our liver.

Become aware of the liver cell.

Breathe to it.

Become aware of the experience of your liver cell.

Breathe.

Let the liver cell experience that you are there.

Let the liver cell experience itself as itself.
Open the panorama.

Breathe.

Let the liver cell experience itself as part of
the community of liver cells.

Breathe.

Now let the community experience itself as a community.

Breathe.

And now let the community of liver cells experience
their part of the larger community of the Whole Body.

Breathe.

Breathe.

~Barry

17

Cell Level Theater

"Matter and form are two principles of things.
Sense faculty and sense object are one thing."

~Meister Eckhart, 14th-century mystic

For our purposes in engaging the body with Awareness (also called: Embodied Cognition) it is practical to consider and play around with functions, or the different jobs a body does, so that you can enter into the theater and work with those functions in a lively way. To work with them, you enact them by becoming them, taking on their role and learning to identify what they do (or would like to do).

For those of you who are not biologists (like me), I am going to give you some acting directions to discover and "sense" your way into higher functioning. By becoming an actor, you can have the embodied experience of the functions required for life. You can feel what it's like when something functions well and when it doesn't.

EJH Corner in his wonderful book, *The Life of Plants*, gives a poetic description of the cell, which is a basic template of life patterns:

"The plant-cell, so astoundingly transparent, minute, and apparently simple, has at the molecular level a complexity comparable with the goings-on of a city. There is the inner city and the government within the nuclear membrane, outside of which lie the streets, houses, shops, factories, post offices, police stations, hospitals, lighting and sewer systems retained by the outer wall; and the lesson is that everything living is built throughout in minutest detail."

We are going to work with a "composite cell" as a template of the very basic functions we need in order to walk around in our living bodies. The body itself can be seen as One Cell with different systems playing together in harmony. When all the systems are doing their part, what these bodies of ours can do is nothing short of miraculous!

In medicine, practitioners are trained to do a "Review of Systems" to assess health. They start with the skin and go through the whole body from top to toe.

You can do that "review" for yourself in a practical way by exploring each system as having a function or a job to perform. Form follows function. If we know what the function or the requirement for life is, a workable solution in matter or form will predictably arise. When we enter into this with our "sensing" and become the object of our contemplation (imagine you are an actor in a play), you become one with it, and then you are participating in the Mystery in a way that can be quite wonderful. You might take a "function per day" and walk around with the questions posed about how that is working in your life.

Barry reminds us to see "how the part relates to and serves the Whole." You know if the trash collectors don't come for the trash, your city is overrun with debris and rats and ugliness. Make sure your systems of elimination is working! At the end of the day, see what came up for you as a reflection on how each part of the system is working for you. Feel free to add questions your awareness wants to explore as an embodied experience.

Warning! For most people, this is way too much information for one session. You may read through the whole section for ideas. The danger is going too much into your thought-thinking mind and not shifting into the embodied experience. Remember: we don't want to separate mind and body, but rather to bring them together. We want to learn to listen to the cells, which are becoming aware. We need to set aside a time to listen.

With the questions I pose below, you can listen to or explore different functions of the cells and help the cells become more aware. So, either choose to set a schedule for yourself to do one "system" a day or spend the next twelve hours going through the Cell City as an embodied experience for all your senses to engage.

Set up the stage as the "Inner City" of your cell. We will use the stage for the different actors to explore their roles. Shakespeare is cheering you on!

Start with the "skin" of your cells, the Cell Membrane. Just as the skin protects the body as an interface between you and the environment, the cell membrane protects the integrity of the cell. It lets things in and out. It contains specialized receptors that detect chemical messages, as well as pumps and pores that regulate the flow of substances into and out of the cell.

In the theater of your life, here are some questions (choose only one to work with):

- What is my experience of boundaries?
- What does it feel like to have healthy boundaries?
- What is the experience of feeling repelled by something? Attracted to something?
- What does it feel like when I am out of integrity?
- What is the sense of being in my own integrity? (There is a "feel" in the body when you are in your own integrity.)

Stand up and become the actor who embodies integrity. Let your body go into one of the questions above. Let the body's movements express themselves. Just let the body lead the way by getting your mind out of the way. Breathe. Move. Allow the body's expression of acting out "Integrity." When this comes to a resting place, feel the micro-movements of your inner landscape, the subtle sensations of integrity that are left behind. Breathe and allow for the experience to stay with you and stabilize in you. You can call it back when you need it!

The Memory/Message Center of our bodies is the Brain, and almost all cells have something of an equivalent, which is the Nucleus. The Nucleus holds the genetic information found encoded in tightly coiled bands (like scrolls) called DNA. This information is like a blueprint that holds your collected humanity and the instructions for how things are made. Requests come into the nucleus to get the right information for a need. These "requests" must travel across a very thin membrane called the Nuclear Membrane. The answer to the request is then carried back across this thin membrane, bringing the information to the rest of the cell. The Brain is like the headquarters of the body, where information arrives from the environment, from life, to analyze, compare, coordinate, and to send a good response back to the body through a wonderful network of nerves that take the information to every organ in the body.

Questions:
- What is the experience of having good information?
- What is the experience of having bad information?
- How do I sense that information is true and practical?

- How do I know when information gets where it needs to go?
- What is the sense of fluid communication of listening and responding?
- What is the experience of good connection (perceiving and responding)?

Stand up and become the actor who will present the role of Headquarters, having a blueprint and being in charge of information (receiving and acting on it). Let your body go into one of the questions above. Let the body's movements express themselves. Just let the body lead the way by getting your mind out of the way. Breathe. Move. Allow the body's expression to reveal its experience of being the information coordinator. Let the rest of the body relax and know that someone is attending to this important task. When this comes to fullness, allow the actor who is in charge to find a resting place. Feel the gift lingering as micro-movements in your inner landscape. These are subtle sensations of good information and good connections taking place. Breathe and allow for the experience to stay with you and stabilize, so you can call on it if you need to.

Our bodies have a foundational structure called the Musculo-Skeletal System. It is comprised of the bones, muscles, tendons, and ligaments, that allow for us to participate in life. Sure enough, in the cell we have the Cytoskeleton holding it all together. There are fine Microtubules that are like little muscles that help the cell maintain its shape. They assist with cell division and help the movement of organelles within the cell and the transport of vesicles.

Let's consider this as symbolic of Structure and Mobility.

Questions:

- What does my structure feel like? Solid? Weak? Brittle? Strong?
- What is my experience when my structure is too tight and rigid?
- What is my experience when my structure is too chaotic or frantic?
- When I feel solid, grounded, and centered, what kind of movement comes from me?
- When I am scared, uncertain, or confused, what kind of movement comes from me?
- What is the experience of moving with freedom, rhythm, joy?

Find your actor's make-up for an exploration of structure. Let your body go into one of the questions above. Let the body express itself through these movements, revealing its relationship with structure and mobility. Just let the body lead the way by getting your mind out of the way. Breathe. Move. Allow the body's expression to unfold. Let all the cells in the body give a standing ovation for healthy structure and responsive movement. When this comes to a resting place, feel the micro-movements of your inner landscape, the subtle sensations that a supportive, grounded structure and responsive movement provide. Breathe and allow for the inner experience to stay with you and stabilize.

Our bodies use all kinds of complex chemicals that are required in just the right mix for every bodily function. We have an Endocrine System that makes hormones, which are lovely light-filled chemicals that help regulate all kinds of functions in the body. The headquarters of this system is the hypothalamus/pituitary (snuggled in under the brain), which regulates the hormones to make sure they're in the right mix and in balance. The endocrine system is in tight communication with the nervous system.

So, if you're really anxious, the nervous system tells the endocrine system to make adrenalin (a hormone made in the adrenal glands), so you can run faster to get away from the saber-toothed tiger.

You could also go through each endocrine gland, which is in charge of a certain area of life, but I'll let you do that on your own if you're interested in that deeper exploration.

Ribosomes, similarly, are found at different places around the cell. They are like little workbenches where proteins are made to serve the needs of life.

Also involved in making other substances the cell needs, is the Smooth Endoplasmic Reticulum that is involved in making fatty acids, steroids and storing and releasing calcium.

Let's consider this function as symbolic of having the right ingredients in the right mix (good chemistry) available for living in these bodies and for all the wonderful things they do, such as creating things, assimilating things, eliminating stuff they don't need, protecting themselves from harm, relating to others and to assessing and maintaining balance within the Harmonic Functioning of the Whole.

Questions:
- What is the experience of responding to a need?
- What is the experience of ignoring or being unaware of a need?
- What is "good chemistry" for me?
- What is my experience of "bad chemistry?"

- What does it feel like to identify what's important to me?
- Do I respect that and align myself with my intentions?
- What is the experience of being in harmony within myself?
- Sense dissonance in yourself and see how your body works to bring it to resolution.

Stand up and put on your acting suit so your body shows its experience of "chemistry," the mix of ingredients being available for different purposes and getting the mix just right. Let your body go into one of the questions above. Let the body's movements express themselves. Just let the body lead the way by getting your mind out of the way. Breathe. Move. Allow the body's expression. Notice how the rest of the body is applauding when this character gives its gift! When this act is over, take a bow. Allow things to come into a resting place, in which you can still feel the after-effect, like micro-movements in your inner landscape. See if you can detect the subtle sensations of having things in a harmonious and lively and responsive balance. Breathe and allow for the experience to stay with you and to stabilize.

Our bodies have a way to take in oxygen from the Great Breath via the Lungs, the favorite organ of the Respiratory System. Oxygen is taken into the lungs, and it is picked up by the blood cells and delivered to every cell in the body.

The cells need oxygen as fuel. If you have ever blown over coals to get them to ignite, you know what oxygen is doing to fire things up in your body. Oxygen is used to fire up glucose to make energy-rich molecules that drive other metabolic reactions. Carbon dioxide is produced in this, but the body can't use it, so the blood cells take it back to the lungs and it is breathed back out into the environment, where the plants (for example) can use it!

The Mitochondria are the batteries of the cell. They use oxygen, glucose and fatty acids to release energy, and they have to get rid of carbon dioxide, a by-product.

So, we might consider the lungs and the mitochondria as symbolic of taking in the Great Breath as the fuel needed to energize the body and keep it fired up.

Questions:
- What is the experience of taking in the breath?
- What is the experience of restricted breath?
- What is the experience of releasing the breath?
- What energizes me (fires me up)?
- What depletes me?

Stand up and let your body show its experience of taking in the breath! Let your body go into one of the questions above. Let the body's movements express themselves. Just let the body lead the way by getting your mind out of the way. Breathe. Move. Allow the body's expression as an actor who breathes. Allow this experience to come to fullness. Notice how all the cells in the body are inflamed with gratitude for the gift of the vitalizing oxygen that energizes them! When this comes to a resting place, feel the micro-movements of your inner landscape, the subtle sensations of having the gift of breath, potent energy to enliven you. Breathe and allow for the experience to stay with you in a subtle but noticeable way, and then allow it to stabilize.

The Heart and the Cardio-Vascular System is a transport system of the blood, the life force, which carries nutrients, oxygen, hormones, and protective immune cells to monitor the whole body. In the cells there is something called the Golgi Apparatus that processes, sorts, modifies, and transports products around the cell and to the surface of the cell.

Questions:
- How is my rhythm?
- What is my experience of things moving around with purpose and strength?
- What is the experience of stagnation, lack of movement?
- What is the "beat" that's going on in me? What does it feel like when it's strong? Weak?
- What is the experience of constriction?
- What is my experience of overdoing it?
- What is my experience of allowing for just the right strength to be available for an activity?
- What is my experience of having "my heart" in an activity?
- Is there any place there's no communication or no interaction?

Get out your costume for the Actor in charge of Circulation to come on stage. As an experiment, see what happens when this actor freezes into one position. Hold your breath. Get tight. Get tighter. When you can't stand it, let go and your body in the guise of the Circulation Actor will spontaneously move out of this "freeze" and re-establish rhythm. Experience the new rhythm. See how all the cells in the body are responding to this rhythm and let them chime in. Keep going, allowing things to come to fullness.

Then get still and feel the micro-movements of your inner landscape, the subtle sensations of having the gift of rhythmic circulation, moving all things to their purpose.

The Digestive System includes many organs. It starts at the mouth, travels down the esophagus to the stomach and through pipes of the intestine, where nutrients are taken in, sorted out for their different uses, and the things not needed are eliminated at the end of the line.

We'll point here to something similar: the Lysosomes in the cells are a little like the stomach in that they contain powerful acids that break down worn-out organelles, digest bacteria and foreign substances. And we have the Rough Endoplasmic Reticulum, which is like the liver in some way, since it assembles amino acids to make proteins that are the basic building blocks of the body.

Questions:
- What is the experience of being nourished?
- What is the experience of being unsatisfied?
- What is the experience when I receive something good for me?
- What is my experience of aversion to something bad?
- What does it feel like when I get rid of what no longer serves me?
- What is it like to recycle things, or repurpose things to find a better form that serves me?
- What is my experience of eliminating what I don't need?
- What is the experience of holding on to something too long?

In this acting lesson you can engage the stage to let your body show its experience of receiving nourishment, assimilating what you need, recognizing what no longer serves you and letting it go! Let your body go into one of the questions above. Let the body's movements express themselves. Just let the body lead the way by getting your mind out of the way. Breathe. Move. Allow the body's expression, playing with one of the scripts you've chosen for it to make visible. When this comes to a resting place, feel the micro-movements of your inner landscape, the subtle sensations of having the gift of food, sustenance mixed with breath, energy transformed for everything you need, letting go of what's not needed or helpful. Breathe and allow for the experience to stay with you and to stabilize.

The Immune System is a complex strategy the body has come up with to protect you from illness and rascally pathogens that could harm you. One of the structures of the Immune System is found in the lymph system, which is a network located throughout the body that is always on the lookout for scallywags and 'ne'er do-wells' who have no manners and must be restrained, retrained or removed. In the cells we find something similar called Peroxisomes, which are a little like the lymph nodes concocting the response to danger. For example, enzymes are stored here that neutralize toxic compounds. Let's consider iden-tification of self vs. non-self, discernment, protection, and adequate response for well-being.

Questions:
- What is my experience of something toxic or threatening?
- What does it feel like when something is helpful to me, standing up for me?

- If something is dangerous or threatening, how do I respond? What does that feel like?
- What is the experience of feeling protected?
- When something is wrong, what does it feel like to say "no?"
- When I have something in me that could harm me, how do I respond?

In your play, invite your body to enact recognizing danger, and responding to take care of yourself. Let your body find a position that it would take on if you were being threatened. Just stay with the threat for a moment. See what response your body has to this threat, all on its own. Experience your discerning body being responsive to your well-being. Liberate it to act on your behalf. Let all the other cells in your body have a parade that celebrate the heroic defender of your well-being! Experience this on your own, allowing your clever body, your astute immune system to show its stuff. When this comes to fullness, allow it also to find a resting place. Feel the micro-movements of your inner landscape, the subtle sensations of having the gift of responsiveness to your true well-being. Breathe and allow for the experience to stay with you and stabilize.

At the center of the Urinary System we have the kidneys, which filter the blood, maintain a balance of certain salts, and remove what is no longer needed by the body to keep things in order. What is removed is called urine, and it moves downstream to the bladder, which is a storage container that holds it until we can "relieve ourselves" in some private place.

The whole cell is filled with a liquid called the Cytoplasm. In this fluid there is a constant ebb and flow maintaining an exquisite chemical balance and regulation all the time. In a way, the cell membrane takes on this role of eliminating and filtering the contents of the cell, just as the kidneys allow for excretion of waste products, removal of surplus materials from the body tissues, regulation of the water and salt content of the body by filtering the blood.

Questions:
- What is the experience of filtering out what I don't need?
- What is my experience of retention, holding on, being bloated?
- What is my experience of flow and release?

Stand up and allow your body to move like a fountain, bringing water in, letting water out. See how your body expresses this fluid movement, cleansing, hydrating, releasing, retaining. Maybe you are a fish swimming or a lake with gentle waves or an ocean storm! Just let your body's water system flow and express itself through your little play. When this comes to fullness, to a resting place, get still and continue to feel the micro-movements in your inner landscape, the subtle sensation still left as your body feels cleansed, hydrated, and restored.

We all have a Reproductive System, which allows us to have children, to make new "selves" to continue on with life. The Centrioles act during the movement of chromosomes when the cell divides to make new versions of itself. The cell reproduces itself. Even if we don't have kids, we all have a creative impulse, the need to bring something new, something beautiful, something of ourselves into the world.

Questions:

- What is my experience of creativity? What enlivens my artistic nature?
- What am I "producing" or "giving" to life?
- Allow yourself to sense your living creativity, inspired by your most unique self.
- Not feeling creative or inspired, what does that feel like?
- What does it feel like to hold back to restrain your impulse to create?

Stand up! Let your body bring all we have done together in creativity. See how your body expresses itself as you contemplate one of these questions. Just notice, let go and allow the body to get on the stage and reveal its secret self. When you notice the expression, when the message is complete (for today), get still and allow the micro-movements of your inner landscape to settle a bit. Stay with the subtle sensation of your "creativity exploration" to be known and acknowledged.

We are bringing Mind, Body and Spirit together: three things participating together as one thing. Can you see how all these "functions" are things of life? Can you see that by bringing awareness to your body, to its tissues, organs and cells, which form a living temple, you are engaged in the Theater of Life, your life!

> As above, so below.
> As within, so without.
>
> ~Hermes Trismegistus, Egyptian sage
> *The Kybalion*

One day, a young boy was brought to Barry's office with his mother. He had a condition called hydrocephalus (water on the brain).

Some little shunts (tubes) had been inserted to help drain the fluid from his brain to prevent pressure, but the little shunts kept getting stopped up.

Barry noticed the boy had brought with him two large grocery sacks filled with toy soldiers. Barry looked at the boy. He looked at the sacks. Then he said to his secretary, "Cancel all my appointments today."

He took the boy into his office and all day long, they set up the soldiers. Barry and the boy, working side by side, sensing and breathing toward the right arrangement of the soldiers.

It was reported to Barry later on that the shunts were draining beautifully.

You see? The theater of our lives is always working itself out.

18

Prayer

When
The words stop
And you can endure the silence
That reveals your heart's
Pain
Of emptiness
Or that great wrenching-sweet longing,
That is the time to try and listen
To what the Beloved's
Eyes
Most want
To
Say.

~Hafiz, Sufi poet and mystic
(1313–1390)

I hope you have noticed that this is a spiritual book. Prayer is a spiritual word and the experience of turning toward the silence where you are moved to reverence … is a good place from which to pray. It is the place of holiness. Because we live in our heads so much these days, it's actually difficult to enter this state.

> "There is a real warning that our civilization needs to hear. If our intellects can no longer close their eyes, if we no longer know how to be quiet, then we will be deprived of mystery, of its light, which is beyond darkness, of its beauty, which is beyond all beauty."
>
> ~Robert Sarah, Catholic Cardinal

A lot of people have been hurt by religion and are very nervous about things like "prayer." Other people are skeptical because they find dissonance between science and religious beliefs that seem superstitious and lead people astray. I know other people who have prayed fervently, and nothing apparently happened.

There, there! I understand this wounding. These are difficult and painful experiences! Ufff!

And, I pray. One day, I discovered "holiness" as a state of awareness, and it became a state I really needed to cultivate, since my conditioned habits are pretty strong. How to access this state of awareness from which prayer arises, "like incense," requires us to enter into … silence. It is really worth discovering. It is an experience. Little by little you get used to finding the silence, to seeing the background behind the words or thoughts, to loving the space in which the bird flies. Once you begin to find it (or more likely get out of the way to experience it), you find a sense that has been described as "peace." Nihilism is scary. Silence is joyful. It feels like freedom. Just so you know the difference. It is a peace that passes all understanding … because it's beyond thoughts. And, you start finding it within yourself, within your body!

You can let yourself experience this peace, this silence and spaciousness little by little. Ah, there it is! Something in you identifies it. Within this stillness your heart is still, but alive and enlivened. Your body rests and can move toward the stillness from which a profound reorganization can happen. Sometimes, I look at a tree and ask myself, "How far beyond the tree is spaciousness?" Somehow, I learned to find it. I learned to sense it from within my body as my gaze went beyond the branches of the tree toward the sky. It is a felt experience. I can experience the spaciousness I see "out there" as deep stillness "in here."

Your mind, however, needs something to do. It loves being in charge. So, sometimes, it can pray prayers. Sensing your intention to heal with love is a kind of prayer. If words come from this, use them like a mantra or a chant. If music comes forth, enjoy it, enter into the rhythm, and breathe with it. If you are moved to say a blessing, by all means, do! These are little gifts given to your mind as a revelation of something that is happening way beyond the mind.

I have my favorite prayers. When I can't sit still, I pray my favorite prayers, some of which have been around for 3000 years, so I trust them. I trust they came from someone more holy than I, so why not avail myself of their power and gifts? I trust that they have lifted other people to healing and grace for centuries and therefore, they have a power that is beyond my own. And, when my pesky mind won't let go, the prayers can take me into the state of holiness.

> Let my prayer arise before you like incense,
> The raising of my hands, like an evening oblation.
>
> Psalm 141

From this state of becoming silent, feeling into the stillness, our whole body's yearning for something we don't know how to name—the gesture, raising of hands; the image, incense rising; the experience of not knowing, breathing and being breathed—helps us know we are in prayer. Every now and then we are invited into the deep reverence of the experience of something very beautiful and holy. Having the courage (the heart) to stay present with all that arises in us, moment by moment, in a state of "not knowing," we let go, and something in that pure silence arises.

> We may think of prayer as thoughts or feelings expressed in words. But this is only one expression. . . . Prayer is the opening of mind and heart—our whole being—to. . . the Ultimate Mystery, beyond thoughts, words, and emotions. Through grace we open our awareness to God whom we know by faith is within us, closer than breathing, closer than thinking, closer than choosing—closer than consciousness itself.
>
> ~Thomas Keating, Trappist monk
> (1923–2018)

When you feel toward your heart's desire (or your heart's ache), and let it come alive in you, it is a kind of prayer. It comes from this very still place deep inside, where you have the seeds of what will help you.

Then can you just let go, and … let come what may?

When you pray for someone or yourself, be still, be silent, and let your heart's desire well up. Sometimes words are given as an expression of your heart breathing into the Mystery. Music may arise, and you can breathe to it. This is another way to experience Cell Level Meditation. You start breathing into the place that needs healing, and you take the breath there like a blessing. "Here you go, little cell, some healing, healing breath for you. Blessings on you. Be well." If this arose from the silence from which surged the deep yearning to be Whole, stay with it. A little longer. A little longer. Breathe! Keep going. Let the Mystery show you the way!

Within the silence
of the silence
Just when you think you can't bear it
another minute
And the ache of longing in your chest
is beyond belief
And the lump in your throat
is stinging your ears
And the howling of your yearning
ends in silence
Within the silence
of that silence
A new heaven opens.

And for the scientists among you, I mention that since 2000, at least ten studies of intercessory prayer have been carried out by researchers at institutions including the Mind/Body Medical Institute, a non-profit clinic near Boston run by a Harvard-trained cardiologist, as well as Duke University and the University of Washington. The results all seem to point toward the fact that "there's something to it." Dr. Larry Dossey has shown the power of prayer to work in double-blind studies.

Dr. Lewis Mehl-Madrona has been working with mind-body healing since the 1980s. His grandmother was a Cherokee Indian, and as part of his fullness he brought Native American healing techniques to his medical practice. He has done research on the effects of prayer with patients who are recovering from surgery. He has found compelling evidence that shows that praying for others can accelerate their healing. Dr. Mehl-Madrona says:

"We're presenting the idea that the brain is a sensory organ for spiritual phenomena. The EEG (electroencephalogram) knows when you're being prayed for even if the patient does not. Medical science seems to be showing us quite graphically that we are all connected to each other and to the larger world."

Prayer

Oh Great Spirit!
Earth, Wind, Fire, and Sea!
You are inside
And
All around me.
My thoughts rise to the air
My feet touch the ground
My cells rally round
To swim to the sound
From Virgin Point to
Gleaming Cosmos
Holy Breath proclaiming
Here I am,
This one being in Being.

19

Conditioned Habits

"I hate television. I hate it as much as I hate peanuts.
But I can't stop eating peanuts."

~Orson Wells, actor, writer, director
(1915–1985)

I love computers. They really show us so much about ourselves, since it was we humans, after all, who discovered the principles that made them work and invented and produced them. Computers are programmed to do many things. In a similar way, we are programmed. Now, if I want to change the programming in my computer, I can't just yell at it and say, "Hey, change the font I'm writing with." No, I have to find the program in the computer, go there, and see what options are available and make the changes. Sometimes I have to get new software! And some things can't be changed, or the computer doesn't work at all.

In a similar way, Cell Level Meditation can be a way of finding the programming and deciding if it is producing my current well-being or not.

What is really shocking is discovering just how unaware I am of most of my programming. Becoming aware that there is conditioned awareness and the body is responding to deep commands that in many cases have not been questioned is a discovery that most people have during the course of their healing journeys. As I mentioned before, it is said that our "conscious minds" are only aware of about 5% of our programming. The other 95% is found in some other "program."

Programming can work in a positive way by using imagination and working with a guided visualization that you or someone else makes for you. These can be very powerful if they speak to you deeply. Many people benefit from these healing offerings. Barry and I have seen people derive great benefit from guided imagery.

And people have asked, "Hey, where does that fit in all of this?" I personally believe that whatever creates a coherent field of awareness is useful for healing. Sometimes, we're uninspired. Sometimes, we're scared to death. Neither of these places is particularly conducive to healing. So, if you have the opportunity to be guided by someone you trust and admire through healing visualizations, this comes to you as a gift!

If you are at a juncture between noticing that your conditioned habits have become rigid and stale but you are not quite ready (or able) to let them go, you may be at an important new edge of your own healing. Our bodies are certainly complex systems.

Most spiritual traditions have some way of telling us that we are challenged most when we are about to make a significant shift. The old adage says, "It's darkest just before the dawn," right? Now, science tells us the same thing that when something new wants to arise, we experience chaos. In fact, in the science of Chaos Theory, after a shift has happened, the chaos (as experienced before the shift) is a predictor of a new level of complexity, of a higher order, that is about to emerge. I say this to comfort you! Even when you feel overwhelmed with the crazy incoherence of your cell meditation experience, even when you are at the edge of chaos, stay present for it, stay with it, stay focused on your intention to emerge more whole, and let a greater intelligence, beyond your thoughts and habits, take you forward.

You know I was a midwife. And over the years of sitting with women at birth, I noticed a pattern. After hours (and hours) in labor, most women would get to a point at which they would say (shout), "I can't do it!". I came to understand they were saying something very true. "They," the woman they thought they were, was no longer "in charge," but rather forces way beyond her were at work for the miracle of life to emerge, new. The identity of a single woman was now infused with the ancient rite of birth, the biological miracle of a body that knows how to birth and the primordial source of life itself, struggling to come into the world. And not long after this intensity of pain, exhaustion and, often, frustration, the baby would arrive. "I can't do it" became the sign for me that the baby was not far away. And then, everything in the room would change into joy as we all welcomed someone very, very new.

Rather than being too worried about being "at the edge of chaos" you are now empowered to stay present with your experience, as it presents to you. Even in chaos, you have the breath. You are going into Unknown Territory, but with your intention and hope and the breath. The rest of it comes from a higher place. More good news—complex systems evolve and order at higher levels of function. By working with the edges of our conditioned habits with awareness, willingness to stay present for what is actually going on as sensation in the body, even stuck patterns are called to a higher level when there is a ripe moment.

Use what speaks to you deeply, where your cells say, "Yes!"
And listen deeply, more deeply, into the silence now for the cells
to let you know about their true and deepest needs, their most
beautiful expression of a Wholeness and loveliness of being that is
their unique expression.

Once, I worked with a young man who was born with cerebral palsy. He had to have surgery to correct severe scoliosis of the spine. It was a very difficult surgery and he had to spend months in rehabilitation. He was used to a crooked spine and didn't really have the "program" for a straightened spine. During that time, we did Cell Level Meditation by phone. He had to recreate new neural pathways for certain muscles.

We connected. Awareness shifted. On my side of the connection, I became aware of the nerve/muscle junction as I was in meditation. Oh! This was delightful! I experienced a sense of electricity being received and responded to with matter; it was a little dance! It seemed like a very joyful interchange. This was already happening in my own body, which I hoped could be a template for his, so his body could "reboot," realign and reprogram. In the meantime, he was having his own experiences: noticing, breathing, and becoming what came to him. He reported that after his sessions, which we did long-distance (good news: consciousness is non-local!), he was able to stand up without pain for longer and longer periods. How much of this was conscious, and how much just happened because of the Mystery…well, I wouldn't know!

"The most beautiful thing we can experience is the mysterious. It is the source of all true art and all science. He to whom this emotion is a stranger, who can no longer pause to wonder and stand rapt in awe, is as good as dead: his eyes are closed."

~Albert Einstein, physicist and philosopher
(1879–1955)

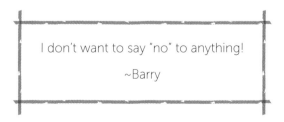

I don't want to say "no" to anything!

~Barry

20

Meditating with Others:
The Cell Community

"I am a success today because I had a friend who believed in me,
and I didn't have the heart to let him down."

~Abraham Lincoln, American president
(1809–1865)

All of the Great Wisdom traditions speak of our interconnectedness. The cells live in community to make the body. Mostly, as I wrote earlier, this community of cells gets along splendidly, with the liver doing its most excellent work, the kidneys doing their wonderful cleansing, the toes doing their tiptoeing, and so on. We have spoken about how each cell performs these functions. We have mentioned that cells, while performing all these functions, also begin to specialize and form a community with other like-minded cells to form organs that are dedicated to a specialty area, like getting blood pumped around (the heart) or transmitting messages (the nerves) or ridding the body of waste (the large intestine).

The organ communities each work in a larger community, which we recognize as the body. What happens when these bodies (each consisting of trillions of cells) come together with other human bodies with the intention of being healthy? When we bring bodies together with shared intention, new levels of possibilities open up.

The Buddhists talk about waking up to the false notion of ourselves as separate from each other. Then there's Jesus, who said it in another way: "Where two or more are gathered, there I am." I take this to mean there is a kind of consciousness there that is different from being alone, and this goes all the way down to what's happening in the cells.

There are potentials for healing that we are just beginning to discover. Imagine: First, I am learning to listen to no-thing, then I am learning to listen to some-thing. Then I am breathing and listening to a dialogue, then I am experiencing this dialogue, and I am surprised at what happens in this listening, this "call and response," this breathing and then becoming. In a similar way, I am listening to "me-ness," and then listening to "you-ness," and because of this, something new arises in awareness, mind, and body.

Perhaps you've had your own experience of the heightened power of meditation when you are with another person or in a group. Someone further down the road in consciousness, awareness, or healthfulness can help shine the light on your own path. Your dance teacher shows you how to turn your foot in a little, and suddenly you can do the dance. Your swimming instructor tells you to put your head down a little, which corrects the position of your body in the water, and you find you can swim faster. Then your whole swim team cheers you on, and you swim even faster and the whole team is thrilled! Even so, as you walk the path or dance the dance, you have to make it your own.

Cell Level Meditation is deceptively simple. It just doesn't occur to us to stay present with and to breathe to the most obvious things that are so familiar we just can't see them. This is where others can help us. And it's also true that there seems to be something mysterious that happens when "two or more are gathered," and you meditate with another

person. A higher energy level seems to be available that may be difficult to access on your own, so you may learn more, come to awareness
faster, transform in ways you don't tend to do when you're by yourself.
One fellow I know said, "I've transformed more in the last year and
a half [by being in an intentional group] than by doing ten years of
Buddhist meditation."

And, as I mentioned, our conditioning is so deep and so much of it is
out of our field of awareness! To help ourselves beyond the blind spots,
sharing this kind of meditation with others can be very helpful.

Kabir, from India, was a 15th Century Poet or a divine "smart aleck,"
as his translator Daniel Ladinsky calls him. He said,

> "The fish
> That is thirsty
> Needs serious
> Professional Counseling."

We are all like this fish in some ways, and our friends can be "serious
professional counselors" because they see us in ways that are often hidden to us. Once, my friends made a comment that startled me, "You're
really intense." They were shocked to realize I didn't know this about
myself. So, I began to explore "intensity." Of course, my humanity of
wanting to please people tried to "correct this intensity," and then my
friends said, "We like your intensity." So, I was glad to be aware of it,
to discover where it was living in my body, to breathe with it, and to
become it. And on and on goes the dialogue, the unfolding, the liberating, the new possibilities, the healing of old wounds, and the co-
creation of a new edge of human potential and evolution.

Since we are each the fish in the fishbowl of our lives, looking for water, our friends can gently say things like, "You look scared!" You can try on what they're saying. Scared? Oh, yes! Where is that in my body? Breathe to it. Become it. And bring your friends along. They'll all benefit.

Did you notice I said, "gently?" We also need to take care with each other that we are not stomping around in someone's tender pain, making it worse. We need to own that we often project our own ideas and issues on others. So, if you work with others, check your helpful heart, and offer what you see in the spirit of kindness … gently. And then, by growing in community we can all learn from and with each other.

By sharing our experiences, and "breathing" with each other, very powerful healings can and do happen. If one person's immune system has already healed from some difficult disease, we now know this is humanly possible. Furthermore, by sitting in the field or presence of this person, our own immune systems can be similarly inspired, primed, and entrained in new ways. We are like the strings of a harp that begin to play in resonance with a note of purity that is sounded in the same room. We begin to hum together.

When Roger Bannister ran the four-minute mile, soon after he broke through the limitation that said, "No one can run a mile under four minutes," many runners began to run that fast and then even faster! In many medical centers, they've noticed that patients get better faster from diseases like cancer if they attend support groups. The principles created in the 12-Step Recovery Groups, like Alcoholics Anonymous, are very powerful in aligning the power of the group for healing.

And, each group also has something like a center of gravity where the participants agree on shared reality. I am reminded of a childbirth instructor who spent a lot of time educating her clients about all the things that could go wrong with them in their births, ostensibly to take their fears away. However, she had a high percentage of women who ended up having cesareans! Somehow, they were all programmed to have things go wrong. So, notice whether your support group helps you move to a higher center of gravity, a higher level of functioning or if it is programming you with limiting fears or pulling you down!

It's also true that sometimes we need to borrow faith from those who have a bit more experience than we do. This is just part of being human. Faith, by the way, isn't just wishful thinking, but rather a deeply felt knowing, usually from lived experience, that something is so. We tune into a basic pattern of being. Of course, if you've had some experience in achieving results at something, your mind is primed and open to repeating the results. Until you've had your own experience, "borrowing faith" from someone who has had the experience is not a bad idea.

Once I invited a Cell Meditation group I was working with to participate in acting out a play, since many people in the group had a hard time with the instruction "to become" what they were observing. So, we used a well-known folk story to practice "becoming" by acting. We worked with Little Red Riding Hood, in which the archetypal characters are all to be found at the Cell Level! We took turns playing out different characters: the innocent (Red Riding Hood, like a sweet little red blood cell was taking nourishment to her grandmother), the villain (the Wolf, like a pathogen, was looking for his own advantage), the Grandmother (the wisdom of lineage found in the DNA), and the

Woodman (the hero, who was responsive to danger, like the immune system, who figured out a solution).

We were all parts of the cell, learning our weaknesses, developing inspiration, acquiring strength and responsiveness. Since we are all actors in Life's Great Play, ever participating from our own natures and gifts, as well as our habits and challenges, in community, we can benefit from group wisdom.

Forming communities of Cell Level Meditators could be an important part of health care in the future, since it would engage our creativity, enhance our growing awareness of the mind/body/spirit connection, as well as make us aware of our interconnectedness with each other, with matter and therefore with our environment. Be the first on your block to start a Cell Level Meditation Group!

The instructions are simple:

1. Acknowledge the Mystery by opening to the vast spaciousness and lovely silence all around you.
2. Tune into your heart's desire to find focus and intention.
3. Notice what comes to you as you turn toward the body, using all the senses (images, gestures, subtle sounds, pressure, movement, vibration).
4. Receive the breath from spaciousness and guide it into the sensations you experience, dance with them, interact with them, be moved by them, and become them and breathe with them.
5. Keep going: noticing, breathing, experiencing, becoming, allowing things to come to the fullness of Your Great Being.

Breath to Body! Who knows what wonderful thing wants to happen through you and you and you?

One final word. When it does happen…breathe to it! Become it! Celebrate! Breathing into gratitude and wonder keeps the Mystery alive in you. If you've been sick, it's easy to get into a rut of how much work is involved in getting better. You have to break this habit too. Take the next breath into:

JOY
(breathe, find it in your body, and become joy)

DELIGHT
(breathe, find it in your body, and become delight)

and

VIBRANT HEALTH!
Yes! Breathe to that!
Become that!
And keep breathing…

Afterword

I went to see Barry a couple of months before he died, and we had a week together – in and out of different states of awareness. I read to him and sang to him and pushed him around his neighborhood in a wheelchair, stopping to breathe with the plants along the way. He would sit in front of a laurel hedge that bordered a park near where he lived, which had a "window" cut in it, and he would gaze through this "window" in a meditative state for long stretches of time. He always worked to find how the parts related to the whole. I don't know what he was seeing in that "window," but he asked to go there every day. He kept saying there was something he wanted to tell me, but the moment never came. His last words to me were, "I love you."

He died Nov 3, 2016. I began a nine-day ritual for him of lighting a candle to pray for him every night. On the eighth day, I went to Mass at a beautiful cathedral I attend, and as I was letting my awareness shift to enter into a state of shared holiness, as clear as a bell, I heard him say, "Patricia! I made it!" That day, the candle burned out. And Barry's work lives on in memory and in love, the kind of light that never burns out.

Acknowledgements

From Barry
(These were his sentiments in life)

For:

- My co-author, Patricia, for her patience, integrity, truth, and joy.
- My wife, Adrianne, who breathes with me.
- My children and grandchildren who keep me young.
- Gene Farley, a wonderful Buddhist, in whose presence I experienced transcendence beyond the cell.
- Dr. Rocco Ruggiero, passionate, always curious, and never not willing, no matter how old or lame, to learn to tap dance.
- All my teachers, too many to list.
- Seth Franklin, a determined patriot, teacher, and quotation collector.
- All those I've forgotten.

From Patricia

For:

- My teacher, Barry, for vast stores of patience, playfulness, insight, and love.
- Antón, scholar, lover of wisdom, and most excellent son.
- Heather Kibbey and Joe Kulin, who encouraged us to publish the book, and who helped make it beautiful.

- Susan Kibbey, Dianne Miller, Joleen Kelleher, and Michael Hawkins who carefully went through the second edition to help bring it to greater clarity.
- My patients and students, who teach me and inspire me by sharing themselves so deeply with me.
- My teacher, Rosa Beléndez, for seeing me.
- My teacher, Richard Moss, who opened doors of awareness.
- My partner, Jim, for standing outside the box.
- All those who have loved me, too numerous to name.

A Few Resources

We are living in times of great transition and new understandings. We are on the cusp of new awakenings individually and collectively about the mind/body connection, and about how meditating and connecting awareness with the body can produce dramatic results. Important research is being done that is shifting our understanding of the material plane we thought we knew so well.

These books have been personal favorites, written by modern pioneers who are charting paths to new levels of understanding, as well as remembering and documenting what a few great ones have known since the beginning of time: the great healing potential that lives within all of us. Be inspired by them and begin to have your own experiences!

Ahern, Adrianne. *Snap Out of it Now*. Boulder CO: Sentient Press, 2007.

Alcamo, I. Edward. *Anatomy Coloring Book*. New York: Random House, 2003.

Allen, Karen Byrnes, and Mahendra Kumar Trivedi, et al. "Biofield Energy Healing Based Vitamin D3: An Improved Overall Bone Health Activity in MG-63 Cell line." *Trends in Technical & Scientific Research*. Vol. 2, Issue 1, May 2018.

Borysenko, Joan. *The Power of the Mind to Heal*. California: Hay House, 1995.

Chilton Pearce, Joseph. *The Biology of Transcendence: A Blueprint of the Human Spirit*. Rochester, VT: Park Street Press, 2002.

Church, Dawson, and Alan Sherr, M.D. *The Heart of the Healer*. New York: Aslan, 1987.

Dale, Cyndi. *The Subtle Body: An Encyclopedia of Your Energetic Anatomy.* Boulder CO: Sounds True, 2009.

Dossey, Larry, M.D. *Healing Words: The Power of Prayer and the Practice of Medicine.* New York: HarperCollins, 1993.

Ewing, William A. *Inside Information: Imaging the Human Body.* New York: Simon and Schuster, 1996.

Feldman, Lynne D. *Integral Healing.* Integral Publishers, 2014.

Gaynor, Mitchell, M.D. *Sounds of Healing.* New York: Broadway Books, 1999.

Hawkes, Joyce Whitely. *Cell-Level Healing: The Bridge from Soul to Cell.* New York: Atria Books, 2006.

Huai-chin, Nan, and William Bodri. *Spiritual Paths and Their Meditation Techniques.* Reno, NV: Top Shape Publishing, 2002.

Institute of Noetic Sciences. *Shift: At the Frontiers of Consciousness.* quarterly journal. These people are at the cutting edge of Mind-Body research!

Kabat-Zinn, Jon. *Coming to Our Senses: Healing Ourselves and the World Through Mindfulness.* New York: Hyperion, 2005.

Leonard, George, and Michael Murphy. *The Life We Are Given: A Long-Term Program for Realizing the Potential of Body, Mind, Heart, and Soul.* New York: Putnam Books,1995.

Lipton, Bruce. *The Biology of Belief: Unleashing the Power of Consciousness, Matter, and Miracles.* Santa Rosa, CA: Elite Books, 2005.

Mayer, Elizabeth Lloyd. *Extraordinary Knowing: Science, Skepticism, and the Inexplicable Powers of the Human Mind.* NY: Bantam Books, 2007.

McNamara, Robert L. *Strength to Awaken: An Integral Guide to Strength Training, Performance & Spiritual Practice for Men & Women.* Boulder, CO: Performance Integral, 2012.

Mehl-Madrona, Lewis, M.D. *Coyote Medicine.* New York: Scribner, 1997.

Moss, Richard, M.D. *The Black Butterfly: An Invitation to Radical Aliveness.* Berkeley, CA: Celestial Arts, 1986.

Murphy, Michael. *The Future of the Body.* New York: Perigee Books, 1992.

Ornish, Dean. *Love and Survival: The Scientific Basis for the Healing Power of Intimacy.* New York: HarperCollins, 1998.

Ornish, Dean. *The Spectrum: A Scientifically Proven Program to Feel Better, Live Longer.* New York: Ballantine Books, 2007.

Pert, Candace. *Molecules of Emotion: Why You Feel the Way You Feel.* New York: Scribner, 1997.

Roizen, Michael F., M.D., and Mehmet Oz, M.D. *You: The Owner's Manual.* New York: HarperCollins, 2008.

Sheldrake, Rupert. *The Science of Life: The Hypothesis of Formative Causation.* Boston, MA: Houghton Mifflin, 1981.

Siegel, Bernie, M.D. *Love, Medicine, and Miracles.* New York: Harper and Row, 1986.

Van der Kolk, Bessel. *The Body Keeps the Score.* New York: Penguin Books; Reprint edition September 8, 2015.

Wilber, Ken. *A Brief History of Everything.* Boston, MA: Shambhala, 1996.

Yakir, Michal. *Wondrous Order: Systematic Table of Homeopathic Plant Remedies,* Book One: *Flowering Plants.* Narayana Verlag, 2017.

Poetry and Quotes

Adler-Beléndez, Ekiwah. *Weaver*. Amatlán, Morelos, México: Ediciones del Arkan, 2003.

Carson, Anne. *Eros: The Bittersweet*. Dallas, TX: Dalkey Archive Press, 1998.

Corner, E.J.H. *The Life of Plants*. Re-published by the University of Chicago Press, 2002.

Evans, Lynnette (editorial selection). *Wisdom for Life*. Secaucus, NJ: Chartwell Books, 2004.

Hirshfield, Jane with Mariko Aratani. *The Ink Dark Moon, Love Poems by Ono no Komachi and Izumi Shikibu. Women of the Ancient Court of Japan*. New York: Vintage Books, 1986.

Hirshfield, Jane (editor). *Women in Praise of the Sacred: 43 Centuries of Spiritual Poetry by Women*. New York: Harper Perennial, 1994.

Keating, Thomas. *Open Mind, Open Heart*. 20th Anniversary Edition. New York: Bloomsbury Continuum, 2006, p. 175.

Ladinsky, Daniel. *Love Poems from God: Twelve Sacred Voices from the East and West*. New York: Penguin, 2002.

Ladinsky, Daniel. *The Gift: Poems by Hafiz, The Great Sufi Master*. New York: Penguin, 1999.

Lopez, Barry. *Arctic Dreams, Imagination and Desire in a Northern Landscape*. New York: Vintage Books, 2001, p. 404.

Mindfulness Study: https://journals.plos.org/plosone/article?id=10.1371/journal.pone.0140212

Oppenheimer, JR. "Analogy in Science," *The American Psychologist*. 2:134, Mar, 1956.

Rumi (translated by John Moyne and Coleman Barks). *Say I Am You*. Athens, GA: Maypop, 1994.

Ryan, MJ (editor). *A Grateful Heart: Daily Blessings for the Evening Meal from Buddha to the Beatles*. Berkeley: Conari Press, 1994.

Sarah, Cardinal Robert. *The Power of Silence: Against the Dictatorship of Noise*. San Francisco, CA: Ignatius Press, 2017, p. 125.

Suzuki, Shunryu. *Zen Mind, Beginner's Mind: Informal Talks on Zen Meditation and Its Practice*. Boulder, CO: Shambala, 2011.

Special Permissions

p. 86 (Ono no Komachi), p. 95 (Izumi Shikibu): Quotations from *The Ink Dark Moon, Love Poems by Ono no Komachi and Izumi Shikibu, Women of the Ancient Court of Japan,* Vintage Books, copyright ©1986, Jane Hirshfield and Mariko Aratani, used with permission.

p. 93: "The Guest House" from *Rumi: Say I Am You* (translated by John Moyne and Coleman Barks), Maypop, copyright ©1994, used with permission.

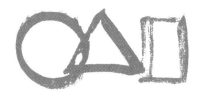

Index

About the Authors

Barry Grundland, M.D.

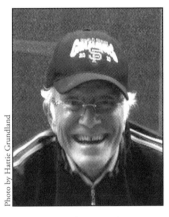

Photo by Hattie Grundland

Barry was born in Chicago in 1933, during the Great Depression. When he was 3, his parents could no longer care for him and he was taken to an orphanage. He told me once that either you became great or a criminal with that kind of childhood. Some of the kids who were in that orphanage with him did, in fact end up in the penitentiary. He was stricken with tetanus during that time, and somehow, during the course of that illness, he discovered meditation and that from stillness (an absolute necessity with tetanus, so the body's movements don't cause horrible spasms), consciousness could travel.

A high school teacher who believed in Barry helped him get into the University of Minnesota, where he studied medicine. He joined the ROTC to help pay his way through college. After medical school, he moved to California to do his residency at St. Luke's in San Francisco. He was called up to serve in the military in 1965, and he became the chief psychiatrist for the Air Force for the next 4 years. He returned to California to finish his residency at the Napa State Hospital. Working with children was a special passion for him, and he went on to do a sub-specialty in child psychiatry.

Barry bought two acres in Napa and had an organic farm where he raised his three daughters, to whom he was always devoted. One of his daughters told me that she knew she could always call him if she needed him, even if he was in a session. He had a wonderful dog, named Snoozer, who went everywhere with him, and he could be seen driving his flatbed truck around Napa with Snoozer, the dachshund, on his lap.

In Napa, he started The Center for Child Development and Psychology for families with children who had developmental problems. He was a pioneer in setting up this center in which psychiatrists, therapists and social workers all worked together collaboratively with the children and their families. Half of the building was for the therapists and the other half was for medical doctors. This was a new concept in the day! He was both director and consultant there, as well as having his own private practice to work with people individually.

Barry was elected to the school board so he could advocate for the support of "the whole child" and look for ways to make sure there were programs for kids with mental illness.

He became very interested in alternative forms of healing and traveled all over the world to visit shamans and healers to understand how they worked. One of his daughters told me about going with him to New Mexico where he met with shamans from both the Navajo and the Hopi nations.

Over time he became increasingly interested in the mind-body connection and worked with guided visualization. This later evolved into the forms of meditation that went all the way into the cells, as well as to working with people in their own unique way. His daughter told me that he was talking about meditation, regenerating organs, and bringing colors to the body before anyone heard about such things. She said that once when she was sick, he came and sat with her and told her to imagine a color. Then he had her bring that color to her whole body and into the part that hurt, and she felt better.

He had a kind of genius that allowed him to "see" systems, whether it was a human body or a corporation. He could see the whole and how each part fit into the whole, and he would help the system see itself. By letting each "part" see itself and how it fits in the whole, the system works better! He told me about working at a resort for a week, and he had each person work in different areas for a day and then another area the next day. People rotated through the various areas of the retreat center over a week, and then went back to their own jobs. By understanding their part (and every part) in the Whole, the center came to a higher level of functioning.

Over the course of his life he would work with all kinds of businesses, corporations, and organizations. Another time, he applied his genius to help a fashion designer come up with a handbag! He understood the times and what women were attracted to that year and so he could bring it together in fashion design. Yet another time, he helped bring together a new perfume, using his talents of bringing the "parts" into a "harmonious whole."

I knew that he volunteered to work as a teacher in residence at Harmony Hill, a cancer retreat center in Washington State. He and his wife, Adrianne to whom he was very devoted, went there for a month, and he worked with 30 people in a supportive way, while also figuring out how to get better funding for the center. The director, Gretchen Schodde, told me that they could barely keep up with him.

His enthusiasm for life was infectious! He could find amusement in a child's cartoon and shift in a heartbeat to an informed appreciation of the great philosophers. He was a speed reader and so he had quite a range of knowledge in many fields. He loved music, theater, art, baseball (the San Francisco Giants), nature, and medicine, and he kept up and stayed current with new developments in medicine his whole life.

He consulted corporate leaders and took homeless people to lunch. Whatever the day brought him, he dove in with delight. His daughter told me he would say, "This is the best!" When she would counter him that he said that before, he would answer, "Well this is the best day now!" He approached life that way. He was present, fully alive in each moment with an incredible repertoire of responses to bring to it.

Whatever Barry did, he was fully engaged. If he loved something, he wore the outfit! He had so much passion for each breath he was given to live.

This text was written by Patricia with help from Barry's daughters, Hattie and Fanny.

Patricia Kay, M.A., CCH, CSD

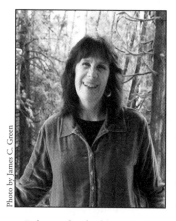

I am a homeopath, teacher, writer, cell meditator, retired midwife, mother, and now, a spiritual director. I discovered the connections between the mind, the body and the Spirit by working as a midwife in rural Mexico for 12 years (along with serious personal health crises and near-death experiences that opened doors of awareness).

I have had the privilege of studying homeopathy under master homeopathic physicians, and I have been working with this spirit-like modality for over 30 years, delving into the intelligent and poetic patterns found behind and within the physical realm. Through midwifery, homeopathy and cell level meditation I have borne witness to the amazing capacity of the body and mind to heal themselves in ways that are often surprisingly creative.

Working with the deep intelligence of the body/mind through meditation was a logical next step in my development. I met Barry about seven months after a very remarkable experience of cell level meditation, in which my foot spontaneously healed, while I was present in a meditative state, "watching it happen." Barry accepted me as a student, and a co-creative process began in 2001 that would find a voice of expression through this book.

Patricia lives in Olympia, WA, and currently works as a Spiritual Director. For more information visit her website:

www.Patricia-Kay.com or **www.CellLevelMeditation.com**

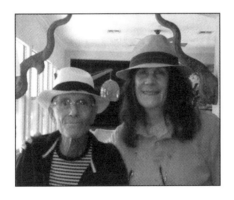

Barry and Patricia
September 2016

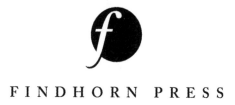

FINDHORN PRESS

Life-Changing Books

Learn more about us and our books at
www.findhornpress.com

For information on the Findhorn Foundation:
www.findhorn.org